Picture Tests
and Short Cases
for the MRCP

Picture Tests and Short Cases for the MRCP

Debra King
MB, ChB, FRCP

Consultant Physician in Geriatric Medicine
Arrowe Park Hospital NHS Trust,
Wirral, Merseyside

WB SAUNDERS COMPANY LTD
London   Philadelphia   Toronto   Sydney   Tokyo

W.B. Saunders Company Ltd
An imprint of Harcourt Publishers Ltd

A catalogue record this book is available from the British Library

ISBN 0-7020-1815-5

This book is printed on acid-free paper

Typeset by Wordperfect, Isleworth and printed and bound in China

Contents

'My method … is to lead my students by the hand to the practice of medicine, taking them every day to see patients in the public hospital, that they may hear the patients' symptoms and see their physical signs.'

Francois Sylvius (1664)

Sylvius (1614 – 1672) was a Dutch physician. He became Professor of Medicine at the University of Leyden in 1658. He was the founder of clinical bedside teaching.

Preface

Many books have been written about the MRCP part II examination. In writing this book I have used many clinical illustrations which may be applicable to both the written and clinical parts of the examination. The clinical slides I have collected throughout my career in medicine, beginning as a Senior House Officer. All patients were willing to be photographed, giving themselves freely to help all those willing to learn, and for this I will always be grateful. Many slides in this book have been contributed by colleagues over the years and I thank them for allowing their material to appear.

The structure of the book has been developed from my experience of the examination as well as many years of teaching MRCP candidates. Many have commented on the nature of the material they would prefer to read prior to the examination. I have listened to these comments, and discussed their experiences during the examination itself, and this has helped in the final structure of this manuscript. I hope it will therefore provide sound advice on the examination, as well as excellent clinical material for the prospective candidate. There is no substitute, however, for adequate knowledge of the subject under test, and the rigorous practising of clinical examination technique. Although there are many who have contributed in some way by sharing their thoughts about the examination with me, any errors that remain in this manuscript are my own. I only hope this book will convey as much pleasure and knowledge as I gained whilst writing it.

Debra King

To my parents

Acknowledgements

I would like to thank Mrs Susan Stewart for her support and expert typing of the manuscript, and the following colleagues for contributing clinical slides.

Dr S. Allard   (Clinical slides in cases 25, 111, 113, 115 and 119)
Consultant Haematologist, Northwick Park Hospital, Harrow.

Dr T. Bayley   (Clinical slides in cases 11, 21, 32, 36, 45, 49, 52 and 94)
Consultant Physician, Broadgreen Hospital, Liverpool.

Dr I. Casson   (Clinical slides in cases 4, 22, 35, 76, 77 and 91)
Consultant Physician, Broadgreen Hospital, Liverpool.

Mr L. Clearkin   (Clinical slide in case 107)
Consultant Ophthalmologist, Arrowe Park Hospital, Wirral.

Dr R. Morgan   (Clinical slide in case 112)
Consultant Physician in Geriatric Medicine, Arrowe Park Hospital, Wirral.

Dr J. Rowe   (Clinical slides in cases 47 and 120)
Consultant Physician, Mossley Hall Hospital, Birmingham.

Dr M.L. Smith   (Clinical slides in cases 13, 31 and 55)
Consultant in Nuclear Medicine, Royal Liverpool University Hospital, Liverpool.

Introduction

This book consists of a series of picture tests. All of the cases are relevant to the photographic material section of the MRCP part 2 written examination. Many of the cases may be encountered as short cases in the clinical section of the examination. As well as explanatory answers to the questions posed, specific advice on examination technique and further discussion of the case is given.

THE MRCP PART 2 EXAMINATION

This consists of a written section, and clinical and oral sections.

Written section

There are three parts: photographic material, case histories and data interpretation.

The photographic section comprises 20 compulsory questions. The photographs may be of clinical cases, X-rays, retinal photographs or pathological material. There is often a clue in the question, so read it carefully. Extra marks can be gained by being specific, e.g. left complete IIIrd cranial nerve palsy will gain more marks than IIIrd cranial nerve palsy. Being verbose is not an advantage and if you provide several alternatives the first response will be marked and the rest discarded.

The case history section comprises four or more compulsory questions. The questions test ability in diagnosis, investigations and management. Often, as in real life there may be more than one possible diagnosis and therefore more than one management plan. This has previously been called the 'grey case' section. The highest marks are given for what the examiners consider to be the most probable diagnosis in the light of the information provided. Lower marks are gained for less likely scenarios.

The data interpretation section comprises 10 compulsory questions which may consist of laboratory data, graphical data, electrocardiograms, etc. Specific questions are asked and there is usually only one correct answer.

1

The pass mark for the written section is 10 out of 20. Sixty per cent of candidates will achieve this mark. A bare fail mark is 9 out of 20 and about 15% of candidates will achieve this and be allowed through to the clinical section where they have the opportunity to make up marks. Therefore, 75% of candidates will go through to the clinical section.

Clinical and oral sections

There are three parts: a long case, short cases and an oral section.

In the long case the candidate will spend 1 hour with a patient and be examined for 20 minutes by two examiners. This is the only part of the examination where history taking skills are tested. The candidate is questioned on the history, diagnosis and management plan as well as the natural history and prognosis of disease. Candidates will also be expected to discuss the social implication of diseases which are becoming more relevant because of the ageing population. Standard testing of urine is expected. Candidates may be asked to demonstrate physical signs.

In the short case section, candidates are examined for 30 minutes on their ability to demonstrate and interpret physical signs in different systems of the body. Two examiners will question the candidate in turn. Usually at least four short cases are seen. Cases may include videos and cardiopulmonary resuscitation models.

In the oral section, candidates are examined for 20 minutes by a pair of examiners. The questions may cover broad aspects of medicine, including applied physiology and pharmacology, statistics, psychiatry, audit, communication skills, ethics and medical emergencies. Candidates may be asked to role play with the examiners, e.g. breaking bad news. They may be asked about recent articles in medical journals and the lay press.

Candidates are given separate marks for the long case, short cases and oral sections. Pass marks are: long cases 4/8, short cases 6/12 and oral 5/10. Taken with a pass of 10/20 in the written section, the minimum pass mark is 25. If a bare fail is the mark in any of the sections then this can be compensated for by gaining 3 extra marks in any of the other sections so that the minimum mark will be 27. A clear fail in any of the four sections of the examination will result in automatic failure. A bare fail in more than one section also results in failure. If the candidate fails badly he/she may be deferred for one examination. Candidates who fail are offered counselling by the college. This will enable the candidate to discuss in detail the reasons why he/she failed.

REASONS FOR FAILURE

Written Section

These extend from ignorance to not reading the question properly. There is no substitute for adequate revision. As well as medical textbooks, medical journals must be read. The question setters, remember, are physicians who keep up to date by reading prestigious medical journals, e.g. *Lancet* and *British Medical Journal* to name only two. Remember that credit is given for precision and the most likely diagnosis. Excessive responses are disregarded.

Clinical and oral sections

Good conduct is essential. The patient (as well as the candidate) may also be nervous and it is mandatory to be courteous to the patient and preserve his/her dignity throughout. Rudeness to the patient and/or examiners quite rightly is not tolerated. Candidates will fail if they are unable to take an adequate history, suggest and interpret investigations and discuss a management plan. Missing physical signs and a rough examination technique will also result in failure. It is wise to ask the patient before examining clearly arthritic hands if he/she is experiencing any pain. Similarly, before examining the abdomen, ask the patient if there are any tender areas so that you can palpate more gently and not inflict unnecessary suffering which may result in failure.

It is essential that examination technique is good. It is always obvious when demonstrating lower limb reflexes, for example, if the candidate is well practised at the technique.

The oral section is about 'thinking on your feet'. As long as what you say is sensible then you should not fail. You could be asked any questions, including ones on ethical issues, and role playing and communication are also examined. Role playing is a valuable way of assessing doctor–patient communication as well as empathy and your overall 'bedside manner', and is being used more commonly. It is in this section that recent journal articles and political medical issues may be discussed. Examiners, therefore, may justifiably test your knowledge of the most recent medical 'events'. Failure may be due to ignorance, not listening to the question or, indeed, not answering the question asked but a similar one you wanted to be asked. It is always best to say you don't know rather than to persist in speaking confabulatory nonsense which will irritate the examiners.

Finally, good luck because, as well as adequate knowledge and examination technique, luck is always helpful.

For further information contact:

Royal College of Physicians of London,
11 St Andrew's Place,
Regents Park,
London NW1 4LE

Tel: 0171 935 1174

CLINICAL EXAMINATION

INTRODUCTION

The most common cause of failure in the MRCP part 2 examination is a poor performance in the short case section. It is essential that you have an examination routine for all systems. This should be practised until you are able to perform 'almost' without thinking. This will not only increase your confidence in the examination situation but will leave the examiners in no doubt that you are well trained and professional in assessing a patient. You should be ready for commands such as; 'examine this patient's cardiovascular system', 'examine this patient's respiratory system', 'examine this patient's abdomen', 'examine this patient's arms/legs', 'examine this patient's cranial nerves', etc.

Your dress should be 'smart' and 'conservative'. There is no need to take anything other than your stethoscope into the examination as other equipment (ophthalmoscope, tendon hammer, sterile pins, etc.) will be provided. It may be helpful though to have a 'red headed' hat pin to test for visual fields and scotomas. You must always be polite to the patient and examiners. Always introduce yourself to the patient and ask him/her permission to examine. If there is potential to inflict pain (arthritic hands/abdomen) always ask the patient if there are areas of tenderness. Do not ask the examiner to explain his/her instructions just to 'buy' time as this will irritate. Also do not ask if the examiner wants you to give a running commentary or a summary at the end of your routine as this may irritate and waste time. You should examine and summarize at the end. The examiner will tell you if he/she requires a deviation from this. Ensure that the patient is positioned correctly (45° for examination of the cardiovascular and respiratory systems, supine with the head resting on one pillow for examination of the abdomen) as far as is comfortable and also adequately exposed (if a female patient, ask if you can remove her nightdress to examine her chest). Thank the patient and help him/her dress and gain a comfortable position when you have finished before turning to the examiners to commence your discussion. If you know the diagnosis, say this and then provide evidence for it. If not, try to summarize your physical findings and the diagnosis may occur to you whilst you do this. For example:

'This lady has mitral stenosis which is complicated by atrial fibrillation and pulmonary hypertension. She has a loud first heart sound and a mid-diastolic murmur. There are no systolic murmurs. Her heart rate is 80 per minute and irregularly irregular. She has a malar flush and a left parasternal heave indicating pulmonary hypertension. There is no clinical evidence of cardiac failure.'

One of the examiners will discuss the case further with you. Do not 'waffle' or veer off into areas about which you have doubtful knowledge as this may provoke a question from the examiner and your ignorance may be exposed. Instead, steer the conversation to areas where your knowledge is fertile. If you have no idea it is better to admit to this: 'I am afraid I don't know the answer to that question'.

There are many courses throughout the country which are designed for the written and clinical sections of the examination. You will, however, get benefit from approaching patients at work as part of your daily routine as if you were in the examination situation. Examining interesting cases in your hospital with colleagues will improve your technique and increase your confidence. The examination situation will then become 'another normal day at work'.

EXAMINATION OF THE CARDIOVASCULAR SYSTEM

The patient should be reclining at at 45° with total exposure from the waist upwards.
Then in turn examine:

1. **Hands** – clubbing, splinter haemorrhages, Osler's nodes, Janeway lesions.
2. **Pulse** – rate, rhythm, volume, character (it is sometimes better to use a larger artery such as the brachial and you must elevate the arm to examine for the presence of a collapsing pulse, but remember to warn the patient you will be elevating the arm before you do so).
3. **Face** – cyanosed, pale, malar flush.
4. **Neck** – look for the height of the internal jugular vein (normal

= 3 cm vertically from the sternal angle). Large *a* waves in the Jugular venous pressure (JVP) are due to pulmonary hypertension and large *v* wave occur in association with tricuspid regurgitation.

5. **Inspect** the chest for scars (left thoracotomy scar, sternotomy scar) and deformities.

6. **Palpate** for the apex beat noting its position and character. Remember you will be palpating the left ventricle, and mitral valve murmurs radiate to the apex beat and thrills may be detected.

7. Place the palm of your hand to the left and parallel with the sternum to assess the presence of a **left parasternal heave**, which indicates right ventricular hypertrophy.

8. Palpate for **thrills** in all areas (apex for mitral valve murmurs, 2nd right intercostal space for aortic valve murmurs, 2nd left intercostal space for pulmonary valve murmurs and 4th left intercostal space for tricuspid murmurs).

9. **Auscultation** – listen for intensity and splitting of the first and second sounds as well as for the presence of systolic and diastolic murmurs. Although certain murmurs are best heard with the bell of the stethoscope, e.g. mitral stenosis and others with the diaphragm, e.g. aortic stenosis, each of the valve areas should be auscultated with both sides of the stethoscope. The patient should also be positioned in the left lateral position to exacerbate mitral valve murmurs and should be asked to sit forward holding the breath in forced expiration to exacerbate aortic and pulmonary murmurs.

10. **Lung** bases should be auscultated for signs of **crackles** consistent with pulmonary oedema.

11. Sacral and peripheral **oedema** should be noted.

12. Peripheral pulses should be assessed as should any evidence of **radiofemoral delay.**

13. Ask to palpate the abdomen for evidence of **hepatomegaly**, which is present with right heart failure. If there is tricuspid regurgitation the hepatomegaly will be 'expansile'.

14. Finally ask if you may measure the **blood pressure** and perform **fundoscopy**. When measuring the blood pressure ensure that the patient is preferably in the sitting position. Use the correct size of arm cuff. Palpate the brachial artery whilst pumping up the sphygmomanometer until the brachial artery is occluded. The pressure at occlusion is the systolic pressure. Then place the diaphragm of the stethoscope over the brachial artery. The First sound heard is the 1st Korotkov sound and is consistent with the systolic pressure. Soon after this there may be an

auscultatory gap followed by more sounds. When the sounds muffle this is the 4th Korotkov sound and when the sounds disappear this is the 5th Korotkov sound and is consistent with the diastolic pressure. It should be noted that most people do have an auscultatory gap and this is the reason for palpating the brachial artery when establishing systolic pressure. Some people do not have a 5th Korotkov sound, in which case the diastolic pressure should be measured as the 4th Korotkov sound and this should be noted. It may be necessary to assess for evidence of postural hypotension. Fundoscopy may reveal abnormalities relevant to the cardiovascular system, e.g. hypertensive retinopathy, diabetic retinopathy, Roth spots.

EXAMINATION OF THE RESPIRATORY SYSTEM

The patient should be reclining at 45° with total exposure from the waist upwards.
Then in turn examine;

1. **Hands** – clubbing, cyanosis, flap of carbon dioxide retention, tar staining of the fingers, rheumatoid hands may give a clue to features of pulmonary fibrosis.
2. **Pulse** – the pulse may be bounding if there is carbon dioxide retention as carbon dioxide is a vasodilator.
3. **Face** – cyanosis, 'purse-lip' respiration (a sign of chronic small airways obstruction).
4. **Inspect** – for chest deformity and for indrawing of the intercostal muscles or lower ribs, assess respiratory rate, look for equal expansion on the right and left.
5. Palpate the supraclavicular and axillary areas for **lymphadenopathy**.
6. Palpate the **trachea** to ensure it is central and establish the position of the **apex** beat.
7. Assess chest expansion by palpation.
8. **Percuss** the chest beginning with the clavicles to ensure you percuss the apices. Percuss each intercostal space on the right then the left. Percuss in the mid-axillary line as well as anteriorly and posteriorly.
9. **'Tactile vocal fremitus'**. This is assessed by placing the lateral aspect of the hand on the patient's chest in sequential areas whilst asking the patient to say '99'. This assesses for areas of consolidation (when it is increased) and areas of collapse (when it is decreased) as well as fluid (when it is decreased). It is a

crude sign and the same information is gained by performing vocal resonance which is more sensitive. This could therefore be omitted from your routine.

10. **Auscultate** – listen for vesicular or bronchial breath sounds and added sounds (crackles and wheezes). Assess for **vocal resonance** and **whispering pectoriloquy**.

The above procedures (7–10) should be performed on the anterior thorax and then the posterior thorax.

EXAMINATION OF THE ABDOMEN

The patient should be lying supine on one pillow providing this is comfortable (no orthopnoea). The chest and abdomen should be exposed. Genitalia should not be exposed.

Then in turn examine:

1. **Hands** – clubbing, Dupuytren's contracture, palmar erythema, leuconychia, spider naevi, pigmentation.
2. **Face and mouth** – pallor, jaundice, xanthelasma, mouth ulcers (Crohn's disease), pigmentation (Peutz–Jegher's syndrome), telangiectasia (Osler–Weber–Rendu syndrome).
3. **Neck** – examine for lymph nodes, e.g. Virchow's node in the left supraclavicular fossa associated with stomach carcinoma.
4. **Chest** – gynaecomastia, scratch marks, bruises, spider naevi, decreased body hair.
5. **Abdomen** – swelling, pulsations, veins, e.g. caput medusae.
6. **Palpation** – ask the patient if there are tender areas. Start in the right iliac fossa and work round in a clockwise fashion with light palpation and then deep palpation detecting areas of tenderness and masses. Palpate liver, spleen and kidneys in turn. Begin palpation of the liver in the left iliac fossa working superiorly asking the patient to inhale until you palpate a liver edge. Begin palpation of the spleen in the right iliac fossa moving diagonally, superiorly and to the left until the tip of the spleen is palpated. The kidneys require bimanual palpation. Palpate the hernial orifices and the inguinal areas for lymph nodes.
7. **Percussion** – percuss any masses or enlarged organs.
8. Examine for **shifting dullness** and a fluid thrill in the presence of ascites.
9. **Auscultation** – listen for bowel sounds, renal bruits, bruits over the liver, e.g. hepatoma.
10. Examination of the external genitalia and a rectal examination are not usually required in the examination situation.

EXAMINATION OF THE ARMS

The patient's arms should be exposed from the shoulders and the patient is usually in the sitting position. The most likely abnormality will be in the neurological system. In turn examine:

1. **Face** – look at the face quickly to establish signs of asymmetry (hemiplegia), Horner's syndrome (Pancoast's tumour) or expressionlessness (Parkinson's disease).
2. **Elbows** – look for psoriasis, rheumatoid nodules or scars which may indicate an ulnar nerve palsy.
3. **Tremor** – there may be a coarse resting tremor (Parkinson's disease), or a fine tremor (thyrotoxicosis).
4. **Hands** – examine the nails (pitting, clubbing, onycholysis), joints (swelling and deformity) and skin (thickness and colour) and assess any evidence of muscle wasting in the hands.
5. **Inspection** – look at the upper arms and forearms for evidence of muscle wasting and fasciculation.
6. **Tone** – after asking the patient if there is any pain in the arms, move them passively bending the arm at the elbow and wrist to assess for tone.
7. **Power** – this should be assessed in the hand, testing the interossei muscles as well as abductor pollicis brevis and opponens pollicis. Power should be assessed by flexing and extending in opposition at the wrist, elbow and shoulder joints as well as testing abduction and adduction at the shoulder.
8. **Coordination**.
9. **Reflexes** – biceps (C5, 6), triceps (C7) and supinator (C5, 6) reflexes.
10. **Sensation** – test touch, pin prick, vibration and position sensation.

EXAMINATION OF THE LEGS

The patient should be exposed from the groin and is usually in the supine or semi-recumbent position. The most likely abnormality is in the neurological system. In turn examine;

1. **Inspection** – look for deformities, e.g. bowing of the tibia in Paget's disease. Look for scars, skin colour and thickness, the presence of body hair, ulcers, muscle wasting and fasciculation.
2. **Tone** – after asking the patient if there is any pain in the legs, move them passively in turn at the hip and knee joints.
3. **Power** – examine for hip, knee and ankle flexion and extension.

4. **Coordination** – ask the patient to run his/her heel down the opposite shin and vice versa.
5. **Reflexes** – knee (L3, L4) and ankle (S1, 2).
6. **Plantar reflex** – Run an 'orange' stick along the lateral sole (S1).
7. **Sensation** – examine for touch, pain, position and vibration sensation.
8. **Gait** – always ask if you can watch the patient walk as this may easily demonstrate an ataxic gait or the high stepping gait of foot drop.

EXAMINATION OF THE CRANIAL NERVES

The patient should be in a sitting position. In turn examine:
1. **Inspection** – generally look at the patient's face for any signs of asymmetry or scars.
2. **Smell and taste** – ask the patient if he/she has any difficulty with the sense of smell. It is unusual to have to perform a formal examination of taste.
3. **Visual acuity** – if a Snellen's chart is not available, ask the patient if he/she can see the clock on the wall or a newspaper that may be available nearby, assessing the patient's vision relative to yours, which is presumed to be normal.
4. **Visual fields** – assess these using a red headed hat pin noting the presence of a central scotoma.
5. **Eye movements** – ask the patient to follow your finger to the right, then superiorly and inferiorly at the right, then to the left superiorly and inferiorly at the left, and then in the midline superiorly and inferiorly. This will assess cranial nerves III, IV and VI and also note any **nystagmus** (VIIIth cranial nerve lesion also cerebellar lesion). Note any **ptosis.**
6. **Pupillary reflexes** – test direct and consensual light reflexes and also the accommodation–convergence reflex.
7. **Fundoscopy.**
8. **Facial movements** – test movements of the eyebrows and face by asking the patient to screw his/her eyes tightly and to whistle (VIIth cranial nerve), ask the patient to clench his/her teeth and to open his/her mouth against force (Vth cranial nerve).
9. **Palatal movement** – ask the patient to say 'aah' (IXth and Xth cranial nerves).
10. **Gag reflex** – IXth and Xth cranial nerves.
11. **Tongue** – Inspect the tongue for wasting and fasciculation as well as movement (XIIth cranial nerve).
12. **Accessory nerve** – ask the patient to shrug his/her shoulders to

test for abnormality of the XIth cranial nerve.

13. **Hearing** – you can test this crudely by whispering and asking the patient if he/she can hear or you may perform Rinné's and Weber's tests.

14. **Sensation** – test for touch with cotton wool and also perform the corneal reflex (Vth cranial nerve).

Clinical Cases

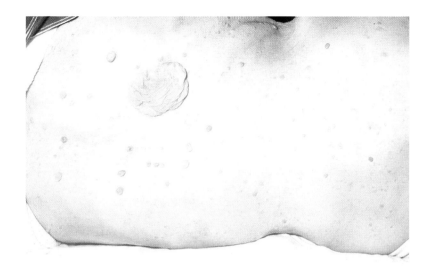

Questions

This woman complained of deafness.

(a) What is the diagnosis?

(b) Why is she deaf?

CASE 1

Answers

(a) Neurofibromatosis (*von Recklinghausen disease)

(b) Due to an associated acoustic neuroma. This may also produce Vth, VIth and VIIth nerve lesions, nystagmus and cerebellar signs and may be bilateral.

Short Case (See Appendix, Figure 1)

Pressure effects of neurofibromas on peripheral as well as cranial nerves may mean you are asked to examine peripheral nerves. Spinal nerve root involvement may cause cord compression, muscle wasting and sensory loss. Other neurological signs may be present due to the presence of a glioma, meningioma or medulloblastoma, which are associated with this condition. When being asked to examine any part of the nervous system therefore, scan the skin for evidence of café-au-lait spots and cutaneous neurofibromas. An association of this condition with phaeochromocytomas (2%) and renal artery stenosis (2%) may mean you will be asked to measure the blood pressure.

Discussion

There are two distinct forms of neurofibromatosis. Von Recklinghausen's (peripheral) neurofibromatosis accounts for over 90% of all cases. It is one of the most common autosomal dominant disorders affecting 20 per 100000 of the population. Its major features are multiple café-au-lait spots, peripheral neurofibromas and Lisch nodules (pigmented iris hamartomas which are best seen by slit lamp examination). Complications include; plexiform neurofibromas (30%), intellectual handicap (10%), sarcomatous change (6%), epilepsy, aqueduct stenosis, spinal neurofibromas, scoliosis (5%), pseudoarthrosis (3%), gastrointestinal neurofibromas (2%), endocrine tumours (2%) and renal artery stenosis (2%). The other form of the disease, which also has an autosomal dominant inheritance is bilateral acoustic (central) neurofibromatosis. This form has few cutaneous manifestations but often has central nervous system tumours, e.g. meningiomas. Lisch nodules are not seen in this form of the disease. Bilateral acoustic neurofibromatosis is linked to abnormalities on chromosome 22. Other features of neurofibromatosis include: lung cysts (honeycomb lung), rib notching and hamartomas of the retina.

*F.D. von Recklinghausen (1833-1910). Professor of Pathology, Strasbourg, France.

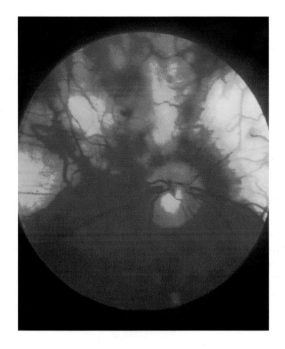

Questions

(a) Name two abnormalities in this fundus

(b) What is the diagnosis?

CASE 2

Answers

(a) Soft exudate, photocoagulation scars, neovascularization and blot haemorrhages.
(b) Proliferative diabetic retinopathy treated by photocoagulation.

Short Case

Diabetic retinopathy is a common short case. It may be a background diabetic retinopathy (microaneurysms, blot haemorrhages and hard exudates) or a proliferative diabetic retinopathy (as for background retinopathy plus soft exudates, flame-shaped haemorrhages, new vessels and accompanying fibrous proliferation, and photocoagulation scars). Remember other diabetic ocular manifestations: cataract; neovascularization of the iris (rubeosis iridis) and glaucoma, neovazcularisation may lead to vitreous haemorrhages and retinal detachments.

Discussion

After 10 years of diabetes approximately 60–70% of patients show some degree of retinopathy. Only 3% develop proliferative retinopathy. Almost all patients with diabetic nephropathy will have evidence of retinopathy. Although good diabetic control should be achieved, control of blood sugar alone does not prevent vasculopathy. The stimulus to neovascularization is an ischaemic retina and photocoagulation using the argon laser prevents this. Indications for photocoagulation include maculopathy, preproliferative and proliferative retinopathy. Maculopathy is diagnosed when hard exudates encroach on the macular sometimes with multiple haemorrhages, or there is evidence of macular oedema (greyish discoloration of the macula). Preproliferative lesions (multiple soft exudates, multiple blot haemorrhages, venous beading, venous loops, atrophic retina) suggest that new vessel formation is about to develop.

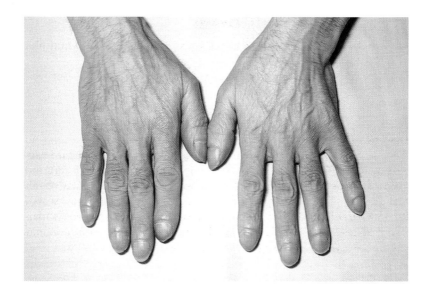

Questions

This man presented with a right Horner's syndrome.

(a) Name two abnormalities in this photograph.

(b) What is the most likely diagnosis?

CASE 3

Answers

(a)   Finger clubbing and tar (not nicotine) staining of the right index finger.

(b)   A right apical bronchial carcinoma.

Short Case (see Appendix, Figure 2)

The earliest change in finger clubbing is swelling of the nail bed due to interstitial oedema and dilatation of the arterioles and capillaries. Test for abnormal fluctuation by placing the pulp of the patient's finger (changes are usually more apparent in the index finger) on the pulp of your two thumbs and palpate the nail bed with your two index fingers to elicit fluctuation. Swelling of the subcutaneous tissues at the nail base causes the overlying skin to become tense and there is obliteration of the skin creases and loss of the obtuse angle between the nail and nail base (becomes >180°). This is elicited by inspecting the finger in profile. Later the swelling involves the nail bed with curvature along its long axis. Swelling of the pulp of the finger results in a drumstick appearance in developed cases. Look for swelling and tenderness of the hands, wrist, feet and ankles to diagnose hypertrophic pulmonary osteoarthropathy due to bronchial carcinoma.

Discussion

Causes of clubbing include-

- Respiratory Disease – bronchial carcinoma, mesothelioma, lung abscess, bronchiectasis, empyema and fibrosing alveolitis.
- Cardiovascular Disease – bacterial endocarditis, cyanotic congenital heart disease, arterio-venous fistulas (usually unilateral) and atrial myxoma.
- Gastrointestinal Disease – hepatic cirrhosis, Crohn's disease, ulcerative colitis and coeliac disease.
- Hereditary – rare, autosomal dominant.
- Thyroid acropachy – may resemble clubbing seen in hypertrophic pulmonary osteoarthropathy (HPOA) but new bone formation seen on an X-ray has the appearance of bubbles on the bone surface whereas new bone formation is linear in HPOA.

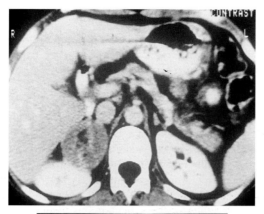

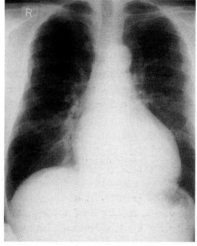

Questions

This patient presented with episodes of pallor, palpitations and sweating.

(a) What is the abnormality on the computed tomographic (CT) scan?

(b) What does the chest X-ray show?

(c) What is the cause of the chest X-ray appearance?

(d) What is the diagnosis?

CASE 4

Answers

(a) A mass anterior to the right kidney.
(b) Cardiomegaly.
(c) Systemic hypertension.
(d) Right phaeochromocytoma.

Short Case

It may be discussed in association with other short cases such as hypertensive retinopathy, neurofibromatosis or thyroid carcinoma.

Discussion

Phaeochromocytomas (tumours of the adrenal medulla) are usually benign and rarely malignant. It can be familial and bilateral.   Familial tumours are associated with multiple endocrine adenomatosis syndrome type II, neurofibromatosis, cerebellar haemangioblastoma and basal cell naevi syndrome. Multiple endocrine adenomatosis type II (*Sipple's syndrome), which is autosomal dominant includes the following gland tumours: thyroid (medullary cell carcinoma, usually secreting calcitonin), adrenal and parathyroid (adenoma or hyperplasia).

Clinical features depend on the amounts of adrenaline and noradrenaline secreted by the tumour and include hypertension (which is usually persistent) and episodes of pallor, palpitations, anxiety, angina and sweating. Hyperglycaemia may occur if adrenaline is secreted. The diagnosis is made by estimating serum levels of catecholamines or urinary levels of catecholamine metabolites: vanillyl mandelic acid (VMA) or hydroxy-methyl-mandelic acid (HMMA). The treatment is to remove the tumour under cover of alpha and beta adrenoceptor blocking agents.

*J.H. Sipple (1930). American chest physician.

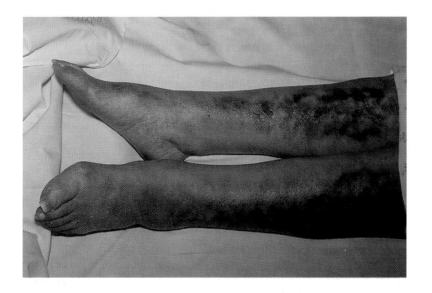

Question

What is the diagnosis?

Answer

Erythema ab igne

Short case

This is a reticulate pigmented erythema caused by chronic infrared radiation. The patient obviously feels the cold and has been too near a fire for too long. Look for evidence of hypothyroidism (facies, bradycardia, slow relaxation of ankle jerks). If it occurs elsewhere, e.g. the abdomen it may be the site of chronic pain that has been relieved with a hot water bottle.

Discussion

The pattern of erythema ab igne is similar to livedo reticularis, which may be associated with a collagen vascular disease (polyarteritis nodosa) or a hyperviscosity syndrome. Erythema ab igne is occasionally premalignant.

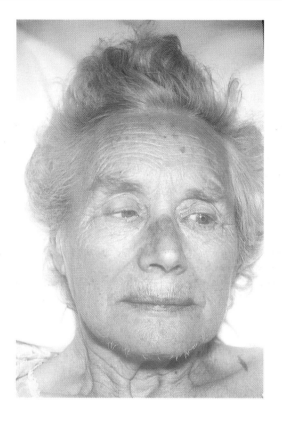

Questions

This woman is looking to her left.

(a) What is the diagnosis?

(b) Name three causes of this condition.

CASE 6

Answers

(a) Left VIth cranial nerve palsy.

(b) Raised intracranial pressure, multiple sclerosis, neoplasm, brain stem vascular lesions, encephalitis, mononeuritis multiplex, aneurysm or meningovascular syphilis.

Short Case

In a short case setting you may be asked to examine the patient's cranial nerves or eyes. If asked to examine cranial nerves this is done in sequential order. Begin by looking at the face for scars or any obvious signs of asymmetry. Then ask the patient if she has any difficulty with the senses of smell and taste. Examine the eyes for visual acuity using a Snellen's chart and then examine the visual fields including assessment for a central scotoma (using a red-headed pin). Then examine eye movements asking the patient if she sees one or two fingers at the extremes of gaze. The false image is the more peripheral of the two and is attributable to the eye whose movement is impaired. Hence by covering the eyes alternately and asking the patient to say when the outer image disappears, the affected eye can be located. During examination of eye movements look for nystagmus and ptosis. Next examine the pupils for the direct and consensual light reflex and then perform fundoscopy. Examine facial movements (Vth and VIIth), palatal movement (IXth and Xth), gag reflex (IXth and Xth) and the tongue for movement, wasting or fasciculation (XIIth). Test the accessory nerve (XIth) by asking the patient to shrug her shoulders. Test hearing (VIIIth) then facial sensation and the corneal reflex (Vth). The command to examine her eyes is easier and includes visual acuity, fields, eye movements, pupillary reflexes and fundoscopy.

Discussion

The abducent or VIth cranial nerve supplies the lateral rectus muscle, which is responsible for eye abduction and has a long intracranial course. The patient has a convergent strabismus at rest when looking directly forwards. There is impairment of lateral movement if the VIth nerve is impaired and diplopia is therefore more severe on lateral gaze.

Raised intracranial pressure causing stretching of the VIth nerve in its long course will cause a palsy and this is known as a 'false localizing sign'. The patient may have papilloedema and other signs of raised intracranial pressure (bradycardia, hypertension).

The causes of a VIth nerve palsy are listed above. Causes of mononeuritis multiplex include: diabetes mellitus, connective tissue disorders (rheumatoid disease, polyarteritis nodosa, systemic lupus erythematosus (SLE), Wegener's granulomatosis), sarcoidosis and amyloidosis.

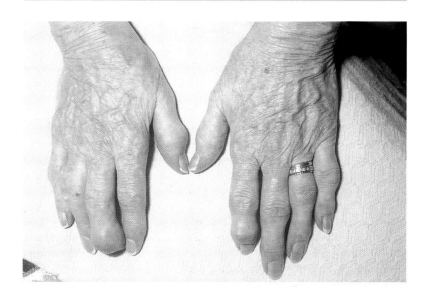

Questions

(a) Name two abnormalities in this photograph.

(b) What is the diagnosis?

(c) Name two complications of this condition.

Answers

(a) Swelling of several proximal and distal interphalangeal joints. Tophi are present on the right proximal interphalangeal joint of the ring finger and right distal interphalangeal joint of the middle finger.
(b) Chronic tophaceous gout.
(c) Renal disease (uric acid stones in 10% of cases, chronic renal failure due to urate nephropathy). Secondary pyogenic infection of joints is uncommon. Hypertension, obesity and coronary heart disease are more common in these patients.

Short Case (see Appendix, Figure 3)

Before examining hands that clearly are arthritic, ask the patient if his/her hands are painful so that you take care not to cause discomfort. Describe the abnormalities, asymmetrical arthropathy, areas of joint swelling and tophi, evidence of muscle wasting or other deformity. The diagnosis is obvious and you should ask to look for tophi in other locations, e.g. elbow, helix of the ears and Achilles tendon. Examine sensation as carpal tunnel syndrome can occur. If the examiner demands a full examination then tone, power and radial pulses should also be examined as part of the examination of the hands.

Discussion

Gout is characterized by episodes of acute arthritis which are at first mono-articular (1st metatarsophalangeal joint in 75% of cases, ankle in 35%, knee in 20%) and then become polyarticular. Attacks are precipitated by dietary access, starvation, alcohol and trauma. Chronic gouty arthritis is asymmetrical and tophi (collections of chalky monosodium urate) may appear close to joints and on the ear, Achilles tendon and elbow in 20% of untreated patients.

Gout may be primarily due to an inborn error of purine metabolism occurring in men and post-menopausal women (men:women, 6:1). It can occur secondary to myeloproliferative disorders, myeloma and Hodgkin's disease owing to increased cell turnover especially during treatment. Other secondary causes of gout include drugs (salicylates, diuretics especially thiazides) and chronic renal failure in which uric acid excretion is reduced.

Radiologically there are irregular bony erosions near the articular margins and tophi may be calcified. Osteoarthritis may co-exist. Uric acid renal stones are amongst the 10% that are radiolucent. Joint fluid contains monosodium urate which appears as negatively birefringent needle-shaped crystals under polarized light. Serum uric acid levels are raised in chronic tophaceous gout if untreated. Treatment is with non-steroidal anti-inflammatory drugs or colchicine if these are contraindicated. Allopurinol is also used in chronic tophaceous gout, chronic hyperuricaemia, urate nephropathy and myeloproliferative disorders under therapy. This reduces acute attacks, blocking the uric acid metabolic pathway. It may precipitate acute gout so non-steroidal anti-inflammatory drugs need to be continued for 6 weeks after its introduction. Probenecid and sulphinpyrazone are rarely used as alternatives to allopurinol and they act by increasing the renal clearance of uric acid.

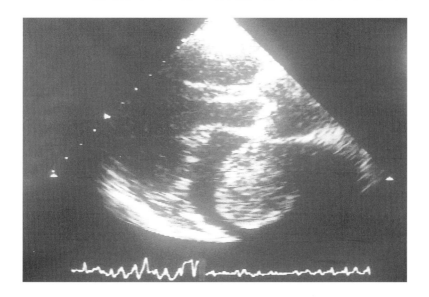

Questions

This echocardiogram (parasternal long axis view in diastole) was performed in a 70-year-old woman who presented with a right hemiplegia.

(a) What two abnormalities can be seen?

(b) What is the cause of her right hemiplegia?

(c) What is the treatment of her cardiac condition?

CASE 8

Answers

(a) A left atrial myxoma. A stenosed mitral valve (image is in diastole). The rhythm strip also shows atrial fibrillation.

(b) An embolus either from a thrombus on the myxoma or in the left atrium or from the myxoma itself travelling to the cerebral circulation (middle cerebral artery occlusion).

(c) Surgical excision of the myxoma is essential to prevent further complications. Mitral valve replacement may also be necessary. The patient should receive lifelong anticoagulation.

Short Case

Examination of the patient's heart or cardiovascular system may be requested. The systemic manifestations of an atrial myxoma are many and include rash, pyrexia, arthropathy and finger clubbing. The clinical signs are of mitral valve disease (even when there is a normal mitral valve, which is more usual than in this case). The patient will have an irregularly irregular pulse of small volume and may have a malar flush. The first heart sound is loud, there is a pansystolic murmur of mitral regurgitation then an early diastolic sound due to 'tumour plop'. A mid-diastolic murmur may follow. The signs may be indistinguishable from mixed mitral valve disease. There may be signs of pulmonary hypertension (loud pulmonary second sound and a left parasternal heave due to right ventricular hypertrophy). There may be evidence of cardiac failure.

Discussion

Myxomas account for about 75% of primary cardiac tumours. They are occasionally transmitted as an autosomal dominant trait although most cases are sporadic. They are usually attached by a pedicle to the interatrial septum. They most commonly occur singly but may be multiple.

Myxomas can manifest with systemic symptoms as described above and may lead to a clinical diagnosis of bacterial endocarditis or connective tissue disease. They may give rise to emboli from a thrombus associated with the tumour or the tumour itself may embolize with consequent symptoms and signs (stroke, femoral artery occlusion, mesenteric artery occlusion).

Operative excision must occur with a degree of urgency to avoid complications (emboli, cardiac failure, arrhythmias). This results in complete cure but recurrence occurs in 1–5% of cases. There is an increased risk of embolization during excision, which is minimized by gentle handling and femoro-femoral bypass.

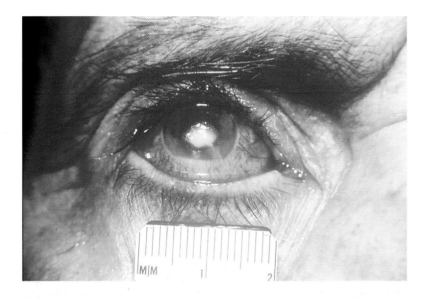

Questions

This man presented with a painful eye of 7 days' duration.

(a) What is the diagnosis?

(b) Name two complications of this condition.

CASE 9

Answers

(a) A fluid level of pus in the anterior chamber of the eye can be seen, which is a hypopyon. This is due to acute iritis.

(b) Secondary glaucoma caused by exudate or adhesions impairing drainage of the aqueous and secondary cataract caused by impairment of lens nutrition.

Discussion

Acute iritis results in a red, painful eye. There may be a contracted pupil as a result of sphincter spasm and distension of the iris with blood. An inflammatory exudate with pus cells in the anterior chamber seen with a corneal microscope is a pathognomonic sign. If profuse, a hypopyon is obvious. Posterior synechias (adhesion of the iris to the lens) are common and anterior synechias (adhesion of the iris to the cornea) are uncommon. The patient often complains of photophobia. Acute iritis can leave permanent visual damage if uncontrolled, may last for months and may recur. Causes of iritis include:-

- Exogenous causes – perforating wounds, corneal ulcers.
- Endogenous causes – this accounts for most cases. Causes are tuberculosis, syphilis, brucellosis, toxoplasmosis, gonorrhoea, sarcoidosis and anklyosing spondylitis.

Treatment includes topical corticosteroids and atropine and a protective pad over the eye. The patient should rest and receive analgesics. Complications may require treatment in their own right.

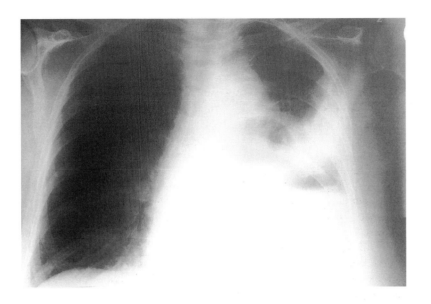

Questions

This patient presented with rigors.

(a) Name two abnormalities on the chest X-ray.

(b) What is the diagnosis?

(c) What is the treatment?

Answers

(a) There is a left pleural effusion, two fluid levels/fluid-filled cavities and an area of consolidation in the left mid-zone.

(b) A lung abscess.

(c) The effusion should be aspirated to dryness and the fluid sent for microscopy, protein estimation and cytology. The patient should receive a broad spectrum intravenous antibiotic initially until sensitivities are available. Chest physiotherapy including postural drainage is also a part of the treatment.

Short Case (see Appendix, Figure 4)

The patient will look ill and have a swinging fever. There may be finger clubbing due to the chronic sepsis or an underlying bronchial carcinoma. The scalene lymph node (the first supraclavicular node to be affected in respiratory malignancy) may be palpable. The patient may be tachypnoeic with reduced expansion on the left where percussion is dull. There will be reduced breath sounds or bronchial breath sounds which may be 'amphoric' in quality over a cavity.

Discussion

Causes of a lung abscess are:

- Malignancy – primary bronchial or metastatic (breast, renal, sarcomas, thyroid, adrenal)
- Aspiration
- Pneumonia – staphylococcal (may follow influenza), *Klebsiella*, *Pneumococcus*, tuberculosis, *Actinomyces*.
- Bronchial obstruction – carcinoma or foreign body, e.g. pea.
- Vascular emboli – pulmonary infarct, emboli from pyaemia.
- Infected congenital or acquired cyst.

Investigations should include sputum and blood culture and pleural aspiration and culture. A bronchoscopy and/or CT scan of the thorax may be necessary.

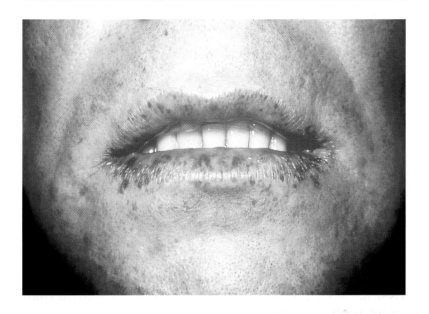

Questions

This patient presented with colicky abdominal pain and vomiting.

(a) What is the cause of the symptoms?

(b) What is the diagnosis?

(c) Name one other complication of this condition.

CASE 11

Answers

(a) Intestinal obstruction resulting from intussusception caused by intestinal polyposis.

(b) Peutz-Jegher's syndrome.

(c) Gastrointestinal haemorrhage, iron deficiency anaemia and malignant transformation of polyps. The latter is rare.

Short Case

There is mucocutaneous pigmentation (hands, feet, circumoral). It is unlikely that the patient will have acute abdominal signs in the examination situation. However, there may be clinical evidence of chronic iron deficiency anaemia (pallor, angular stomatitis, glossitis and koilonychia).

Discussion

Peutz-Jegher's syndrome is mucocutaneous pigmentation and gastrointestinal polyposis. It is inherited as an autosomal dominant trait. The polyps may occur anywhere in the gastrointestinal tract and they are hamartomas. Small intestinal polyps may cause intussusception resulting in intestinal obstruction and may require bowel resection. Definite association with malignancy is rare but may occur in the gastroduodenal region. Gastroduodenal and colonic polyps may also cause anaemia and are easily removed by endoscopic snare polypectomy.

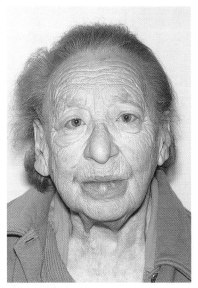 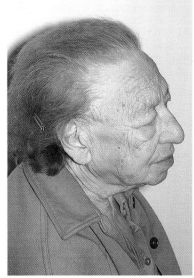

Questions

This 80-year-old woman complained of constipation and paraesthesia in both hands.

(a) Name two physical signs.

(b) What is the cause of her paraesthesiae?

(c) What is the diagnosis?

(d) Name two abnormalities she may have on her ECG.

Answers

(a) There is periorbital oedema, diffuse alopoecia and a pale ('peaches and cream') complexion.

(b) Bilateral carpal tunnel syndrome.

(c) Hypothyroidism.

(d) Sinus bradycardia, low voltage complexes, flattened or inverted T waves. If she also has hypothermia (which is a rare presentation), J waves (at junction of QRS complex and ST segment) may be present.

Short Case (see Appendix, Figure 5)

The patient may be overweight and have typical myxoedematous facies (thickened, coarse facial features with periorbital puffiness). The skin is pale (due to anaemia which may be normochromic or macrocytic) and has a yellowish tint (due to carotenaemia) resulting in the so-called 'peaches and cream' complexion. The skin is dry and rough and there is non-pitting swelling of the subcutaneous tissues due to deposition of mucopolysaccharides. The patient may be deaf with a hoarse, croaky voice. The hair is thin and brittle. The pulse is slow (sinus bradycardia) and may be irregular (atrial fibrillation) owing to associated ischaemic heart disease. There may be a goitre if hypothyroidism is secondary to *Hashimoto's thyroiditis. The patient is slow mentally (dementia, myxoedema madness) and physically and there is slow relaxation of the ankle jerks (myotonia). Other neurological manifestations include carpal tunnel syndrome, peripheral neuropathy, cerebellar ataxia and epilepsy.

Discussion

Hypothyroidism may present as Hashimoto's disease (autoimmune thyroiditis) when there is a goitre or as primary hypothyroidism if the gland atrophies without producing a goitre. Circulating thyroid antibodies are present. Other causes of hypothyroidism include iatrogenic (after radioiodine for thyrotoxicosis or destructive therapy for thyroid carcinoma, antithyroid drugs), primary agenesis (cretinism) and hypopituitarism.

There is often a family history of thyroid disease or other associated autoimmune diseases that may co-exist, e.g. pernicious anaemia (10% of cases), *Graves' disease, *Addison's disease, systemic lupus erythematosus, diabetes mellitus, rheumatoid disease, primary ovarian failure or hypoparathyroidism.

As well as the symptoms above, the patient may complain of cold intolerance, constipation, menorrhagia and angina (this may be precipitated by treatment with thyroxine which should be prescribed in low doses initially especially in the elderly).

The treatment is lifelong thyroxine, 25–300 µg daily beginning with low doses and increasing by 25 µg increments every 14 days.

*H. Hashimoto (1881–1934) Japanese surgeon.
*R.J. Graves (1797–1853) Irish physician.
*J. Addison (1793–1860) English physician.

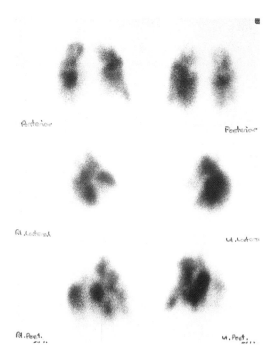

Anterior

Posterior

Rt .Lateral

Lt .Lateral

Rt .Post.

Lt .Post.

Questions

This patient presented with a sudden onset of breathlessness. She had been suffering from diarrhoea for 2 months and had lost 10 kg in weight.

(a) What does her perfusion lung scan show?

(b) What is the cause of her breathlessness?

(c) Name three abnormalities that may be present on her ECG.

(d) What is the most likely cause of her gastrointestinal symptoms?

Answers

(a)   Multiple perfusion defects especially on the right.
(b)   Multiple pulmonary emboli.
(c)   Right ventricular strain (right bundle branch block, inverted T waves in leads V1 to V4), sinus tachycardia, S1 Q3 T3 pattern, and atrial fibrillation.
(d)   A colonic carcinoma.

Short Case

The patient may have signs of a deep vein thrombosis. The patient may be breathless with a rapid pulse, a low blood pressure and a raised jugular venous pressure (JVP). There may be central cyanosis. Examination of the chest may reveal signs of an associated pleural effusion.

Discussion

Pulmonary emboli result from thrombosis of the pelvic or deep leg veins. Causes include:

- Following surgery (10 days classically).
- Venous stasis – prolonged bed rest, heart failure, stroke.
- Increased coagulability – malignancy, oral contraceptives, polycythaemia.

The symptoms include breathlessness, pleuritic pain, haemoptysis and collapse as a result of circulatory failure. A chest X-ray may show an area of oligaemia, a dilated pulmonary artery, areas of segmental collapse (atelectasis), a pleural effusion or, indeed, may be normal. ECG changes occur with larger emboli and are listed above. Blood gases show type I respiratory failure (a low $P\text{CO}_2$ and $P\text{O}_2$)

Treatment is full anticoagulation (intravenous heparin for 5 days and warfarin for 6 months) and correction of the underlying cause where possible. With massive pulmonary emboli, thrombolysis and/or operative removal with bypass surgery may be necessary.

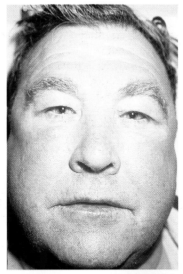

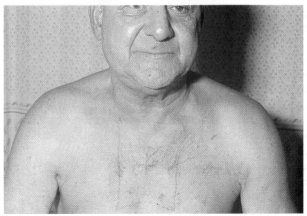

Questions

These two men have the same disease.

(a) Name two abnormalities in the man's face.

(b) Name two abnormalities on the man's chest.

(c) What is the cause of these signs?

(d) Name the most likely underlying diagnosis.

Answers

(a) The face is oedematous and there are subconjunctival haemorrhages caused by increased venous pressure.

(b) Prominent veins and ink marks from radiotherapy treatment.

(c) Superior vena cava obstruction.

(d) Bronchial carcinoma (compression may be due to the tumour itself or involved lymph nodes).

Short Case

The patient may be breathless and have stridor. There may be finger clubbing and tar staining of the fingers. The face and upper extremities are oedematous, neck and chest veins are prominent and there is conjunctival oedema/haemorrhages. There may be specific chest signs resulting from a bronchial carcinoma: collapse, effusion, consolidation and supraclavicular lymph nodes.

Discussion

As well as bronchial carcinoma, other causes of superior vena cava obstruction are mediastinal goitre or fibrosis, lymphoma and aortic aneurysm. The patient complains of headaches exacerbated by coughing and may have dysphagia, breathlessness, dizziness and blackouts. Treatment with radiotherapy is effective. Superior vena caval stents inserted under radiographic control usually relieve symptoms and signs. They are expensive but effective.

- Non pulsatile distension of NK. V.
- Dilated anastomotic V. on chest wall
- CT together c MRI are investi. of choice for mediast. tumours.

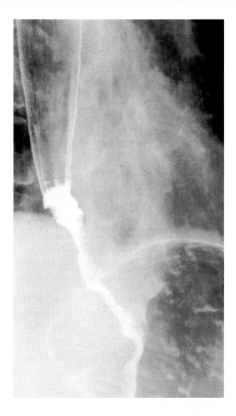

Questions

This 63-year-old man complained of dysphagia.

(a) What is the diagnosis?

(b) Name two other symptoms he may have.

Answers

(a)   Oesophageal carcinoma. This barium swallow shows a long irregular stricture in the lower third of the oesophagus.

(b)   Weight loss, regurgitation and pain (late symptom).

Short Case

The patient is cachectic and may have supraclavicular lymph nodes and an epigastric mass because of involvement of the fundus of the stomach. There may be hepatomegaly from metastatic spread.

Discussion

Carcinoma of the oesophagus is more common in men (3:1). It is more common in Japan and occurs at a younger age than in Western countries. It may be squamous cell or adenocarcinoma. The latter occurs more commonly in the lower third of the oesophagus where it may be secondary to carcinoma of the stomach, and the former occurs more commonly in the middle third. In women the neoplasm is most commonly in the upper third of the oesophagus.

Dysphagia is unpleasant and treatment is by operative resection, radiotherapy and/or palliative procedures. The latter consists of insertion of a tube (Celestin, Atkinson) or insertion of an expandable stent (this is being used more often).

The overall 5-year survival is 10%. Most cases are inoperable at presentation and combined treatments (radiotherapy and surgery) are little better than either alone.

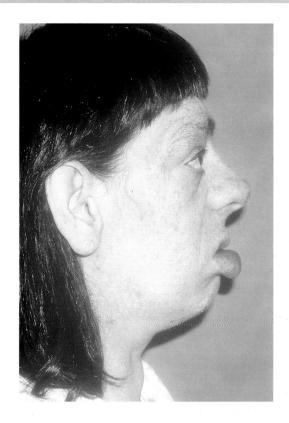

Questions

(a) Name three physical signs in this photograph.

(b) What is the diagnosis?

(c) What is the cause of this condition?

(d) Name two symptoms she may have.

CASE 16

Answers

(a) Prominent supraorbital ridges, large nose, large ear, large protruding lower lip and goitre.

(b) Acromegaly.

(c) Excessive secretion of growth hormone from a pituitary adenoma (usually eosinophil cells).

(d) Excessive sweating, acne, greasy skin, increasing size of shoes, gloves, hats, etc., paraesthesia of hands (carpal tunnel syndrome), arthralgia, headache, visual field or acuity disturbance, amenorrhoea and decreased libido (hypogonadism), galactorrhoea, polyuria and polydipsia (diabetes mellitus, hypercalcaemia, diabetes insipidus).

Short Case (see Appendix, Figures 6–8)

The patient has a typical facial appearance, as described, owing to enlargement of bones and soft tissues. Hands and feet are large and shaking the hand feels like losing your hand in dough. There may be signs of carpal tunnel syndrome. There is macroglossia. The patient is hirsute and has a husky voice. There is a bitemporal hemianopia. The patient may be hypertensive (15% of cases) and have signs resulting from cardiomyopathy (congestive heart failure). There may be signs resulting from diabetes mellitus (retinopathy, peripheral neuropathy) (10% of cases).

Discussion

The mean age at presentation is 40 years. Onset is usually 14 years prior to presentation indicating the slow insidious effects of excessive growth hormone. There is enlargement of soft tissues, bones and viscera.

Investigations will reveal a high level of circulating growth hormone not suppressed by glucose in a standard glucose tolerance test. A skull X-ray may show sella enlargement, large supraorbital ridges and a protruding lower jaw. A CT scan of the head reveals the tumour and will demonstrate suprasellar extension. X-rays of the hands and feet show tufting of the terminal phalanges. A chest X-ray and ECG may show evidence of left ventricular hypertrophy.

Life expectancy is reduced owing to the cardiovascular complications (heart failure, arrhythmias). Trans-sphenoidal hypophysectomy is the treatment of choice but craniotomy is sometimes needed if there is suprasellar extension of the tumour. Yttrium implants and external irradiation are alternatives to surgery but have their own complications: damage to optic tracts, diabetes insipidus and aseptic bone necrosis. Octreotide by subcutaneous injection can be used in the short or long term. Bromocriptine, which reduces growth hormone and prolactin levels, may be used as an adjunct or as sole therapy in those not fit for other treatments.

48

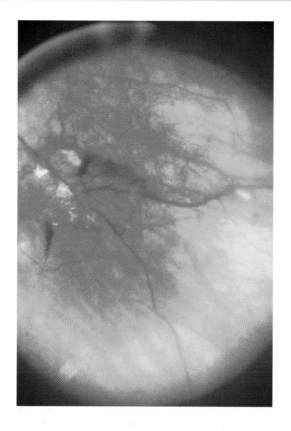

Questions

This patient had a deformed painless ankle.

(a) Name two abnormalities in this photograph.

(b) What is the diagnosis?

(c) What is the cause of the ankle abnormality?

CASE 17

Answers

(a) New vessels, flame-shaped haemorrhage, hard and soft exudates.
(b) Proliferative diabetic retinopathy.
(c) Neuropathic joint (*Charcot's joint).

Short Case (See Case 2)

The ankle joint will be deformed and swollen and may have an abnormal range of movement which is painless. Examine for peripheral neuropathy and neuropathic ulcers. There may also be evidence of peripheral vascular disease.

Discussion

A Charcot's joint (neuropathic joint) results in gross deformity, osteoarthrosis and new bone formation from repeated trauma. Causes of neuropathy joint include; diabetes mellitus, tabes dorsalis, syringomyelia, leprosy, hereditary neuropathies (Charcot-Marie-Tooth disease) and neurofibromatosis (from pressure on sensory nerve roots).

*J.M. Charcot (1825–1893). French physician.

- Pathogenesis — Altered bld flow secondary to impaired Sympathetic control.

- Predisposing ds. — • Diab neuropathy) ankle
              • Syringomyelia ↓
              Shoulder, elbow, wrist

✓ P/w chronic monoarthritis / dislocation.
        • Leprosy (hands, feet)

• Compli. by periph. Nv. entrapment & Sp. cord compr.
        • Tabes dorsalis (knee, spine)

- Xray — Gross loss of cart. & bone c disorg. of Ⓝ architecture & often multi loose bodies & either +

50

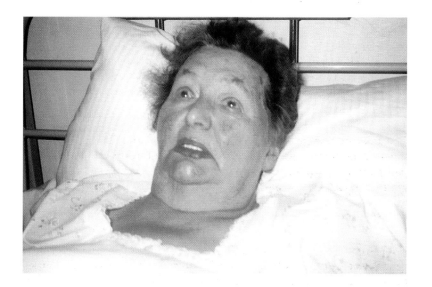

Questions

This woman presented with sudden onset of fever, headache and myalgia. Her urea was 34 mmol/l and creatinine 500 µmol/l. She was an enthusiast of country walks and had had several 'tic' bites from walking in the Yorkshire Dales 2 weeks previously.

(a) What physical sign is demonstrated?

(b) What is the diagnosis?

(c) What is the treatment?

Answers

(a) Jaundice.
(b) *Weil's disease (leptospirosis, icterohaemorrhagiae).
(c) Treatment is mainly supportive for renal and hepatic failure. Penicillin and tetracycline are effective in the early stages.

Short case

Unlikely to be seen as a short case. The patient is jaundiced with a fever and has conjunctival suffusion/haemorrhages. There may be a haemorrhage tendency (bruising) and meningeal irritation (neck stiffness). Myocarditis may result in signs of cardiac failure. There will be protein, red and white cells and casts in the urine as evidence of nephritis.

Discussion

There are about 50 cases of leptospirosis in Britain each year with about three deaths from renal and cardiac failure. The infection is more common in the summer because of farming and leisure activities. The organism Leptospira icterohaemorrhagiae is carried by rats and is transmitted to man directly in the urine of infected rats or via contaminated water through skin abrasions or mucous membranes.

The incubation period is about 10 days. Hepatitis, myocarditis and nephritis are the main features with a tendency to bleed as a result of inflammation of the capillaries. The illness is worse on the 14th day and this is when deaths are most likely. Recovery is usually complete.

*P.S.A. Weil (1848–1916). German physician.

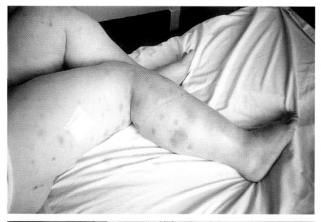

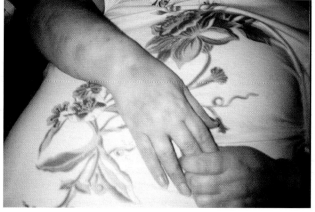

Questions

This 34-year-old woman complained of sore throat of 3 days'
duration.

(a) What is the diagnosis?

(b) What is the cause?

(c) Name three other causes of this condition.

(d) What is the treatment?

Answers

(a) Erythema nodosum.

(b) Streptococcal sore throat.

(c) Sarcoidosis, tuberculosis, drugs (salicylates, oral contraceptives, penicillin, sulphonamides), ulcerative colitis, Crohn's disease, pregnancy, syphilis, *Behçet's disease, toxoplasmosis, leprosy, rheumatic fever and idiopathic.

(d) Treat the underlying cause (oral penicillin or erythromycin if allergic to penicillin, as in this case). The pain and swelling of the lesions are treated symptomatically with non-steroidal anti-inflammatory drugs.

Short Case (see Appendix, Figure 9)

If associated with sarcoidosis there may be features of this: arthralgia, generalized lymphadenopathy, lupus pernio, dyspnoea, parotitis, hepatosplenomegaly, peripheral neuropathy and cranial nerve lesions. If associated with Behçet's disease there may be evidence of oral and genital ulceration, thrombophlebitis, arthralgia of large joints, iritis and neurological manifestations such as myelitis.

Discussion

Raised, red, tender lesions (these pass through the changes of a bruise with healing) of erythema nodosum are more common in females and occur most commonly on the shins but can occur anywhere on the body. There is subcutaneous inflammation and a vasculitis. Resolution is complete but it may recur.

*H. Behçet (1889–1948). Turkish dermatologist.

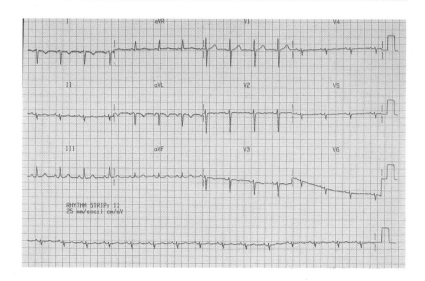

Questions

This is the ECG of an overweight 40-year-old woman who presented with left hypochondrial pain, fever and vomiting. She had a scar in her left iliac fossa.

(a) What is the diagnosis on the ECG?

(b) What is the cause of her symptoms?

(c) What is the likely reason for her abdominal scar?

(d) What is the reason for all the above?

Answers

(a) Dextrocardia. The limb leads are exactly as if the arm leads are transposed. In the chest leads the QRS complexes reduce in size from V1 to V6 as the electrode moves away from the bulk of the left ventricle.
(b) Acute cholecystitis.
(c) Appendicectomy scar.
(d) Situs inversus.

Short case

Examination of the cardiovascular system should be normal except the apex beat is not palpated on the left but is in the right 5th intercostal space. If dextrocardia is associated with *Kartagener's syndrome (dextrocardia, bronchiectasis, situs inversus, infertility, sinusitis, otitis media), then examination of the chest may reveal signs relevant to bronchiectasis (crackles, wheezes, collapse, consolidation). Ask to examine the abdomen to establish which side the liver is on.

Discussion

In situs inversus all the thoracic and abdominal viscera are transposed. The left lung has three lobes and the right has two. The liver is on the left and the gastric fundus on the right. The patient is otherwise normal. Dextrocardia without evidence of situs inversus is usually associated with cardiac malformation. It may occur with cardiac malformation in Turner's syndrome (coarctation of the aorta, atrial septal defect, ventricular septal defect, aortic stenosis).

*M. Kartagener. Swiss physician.

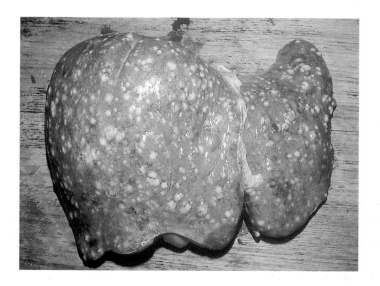

Questions

(a) What does this pathological specimen show?

(b) Give two possible underlying causes.

Answers

(a)   Multiple metastatic deposits in the liver.

(b)   The most likely cause is spread via the circulation from the bowel, e.g. colonic carcinoma, stomach carcinoma, but almost any tumour may metastasize to the liver.

Short Case

The patient with liver metastases will be cachectic, jaundiced and may have evidence of bleeding (bruises) as a result of abnormal liver function. Supraclavicular nodes may be present (*Virchow's nodes, *Troisier's sign – left supraclavicular lymph nodes involved from carcinoma of stomach). Abdominal examination will reveal an enlarged knobbly liver which is usually non-tender. There may be evidence of a primary tumour (mass in left iliac fossa) or ascites.

Discussion

The most common liver tumours are due to secondary spread. Any tumour can metastasize to the liver by blood-borne spread. Primary malignant tumours can metastasize within the liver and give the appearance shown, as can some rare benign primary liver tumours such as cholangioadenomas. Liver tumours can be classified as follows:

- **Primary benign** – haemangioma (usually solitary), hepatoadenomas, cholangioadenomas (may resemble metastases).
- **Primary malignant** – hepatoma (usually occurs secondary to cirrhosis and affects about 20% of cases), cholangiocarcinoma, angiosarcoma.
- **Secondary malignant** – carcinoma (spread from any primary tumour), lymphoma, carcinoid (spread to liver gives rise to carcinoid syndrome).

*R.L.K. Virchow (1821–1902). German professor of pathology.

*C.E. Troisier (1844–1919). French pathologist.

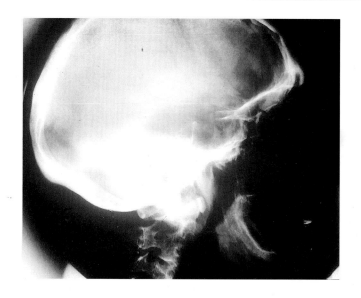

Questions

(a) What is the abnormality on this skull X-ray?

(b) What is the cause?

Answers

(a)   An enlarged pituitary fossa.

(b)   A pituitary tumour.

Short Case

Local pressure from the tumour in the optic tracts causes visual field defects, classically bitemporal hemianopia (upper temporal field defects occur first). There is a decrease in visual acuity which must be assessed. Long-standing pressure causes optic atrophy. Lateral extension of the tumour into the cavernous sinus can cause IIIrd, IVth and VIth cranial nerve palsies.

Other clinical signs depend on the nature of the tumour; acromegaly (see case 16), hypopituitarism (chromophobe adenoma, loss of body hair, pallor and skin depigmentation, signs of hypothyroidism and hypoadrenalism), prolactinoma (usually a microadenoma of the chromophobe type causing galactorrhoea and gynaecomastia), Cushing's disease (basophil adenoma, moon face, 'buffalo' hump, proximal myopathy, striae, kyphosis from osteoporotic vertebral collapse, hirsutism, acne, hypertension).

Discussion

Pituitary tumours are almost always benign and may arise from the anterior or posterior pituitary or remnants of the craniopharyngeal pouch. Pituitary tumours account for 10% of clinically significant intracranial neoplasms. Chromophobe adenomas are the most common type and are usually the largest tumours. They may be part of the multiple endocrine adenomatosis (MEA) syndrome type I (*Wermer's syndrome, autosomal dominant) associated with other endocrine tumours (parathyroid, pancreatic islets, adrenal cortex, thyroid) when the pituitary tumour is usually a prolactinoma. Pituitary tumours can be classified as follows:

- Anterior pituitary
  - Functioning: prolactin secreting, growth hormone secreting, adrenocorticotropic hormone (ACTH) secreting, thyroid-stimulating hormone (TSH) or gonadatrophin secreting (rare).
  - Non functioning: chromophobe adenoma, sarcoma.
- Posterior pituitary
  - craniopharyngioma
  - ganglioneuroma
  - astrocytoma (rare)

*P. Wermer. American physician

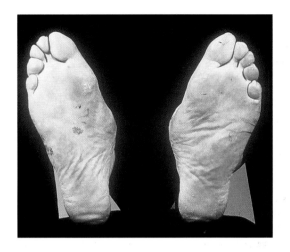

Questions

(a) Name two abnormalities in this photograph.

(b) What is the diagnosis?

Answers

(a)   Deformity resulting from subluxation of the talus bilaterally, and ulceration on the plantar aspect of the right foot.

(b)   Charcot's (neuropathic) arthropathy and neuropathic ulcers resulting from diabetes mellitus (most likely).

Short Case

Examine for peripheral neuropathy and other signs of diabetes mellitus (retinopathy). Neuropathic joints occur in a minority of patients with diabetes mellitus.

Discussion

Other causes of neuropathic joints include syringomyelia, tabes dorsalis, etc. (see case 17).

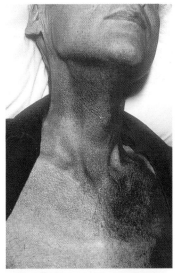

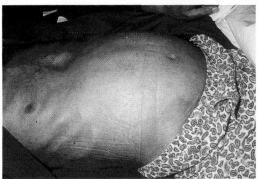

Questions

This 70-year-old man presented with episodic diarrhoea. He had hepatomegaly and signs of pulmonary stenosis.

(a) Name two physical signs that can be seen.

(b) What other heart valve may be abnormal?

(c) What has caused his symptoms and signs?

(d) What is the diagnosis?

Answers

(a) Flushing (neck and chest area), raised jugular venous pressure, cachexia and ascites.

(b) Tricuspid valve (usually regurgitation but stenosis can occur).

(c) Secretion of 5-hydroxytryptamine (serotonin) and kinin peptides.

(d) Carcinoid syndrome

Short Case

During a paroxysm there will be visible flushing of the skin, predominantly of the head and neck but also of the trunk with a rise in skin temperature and associated facial oedema in severe cases. The patient may be breathless and there is bronchospasm. There is a tachycardia and a low systolic blood pressure. The patient is usually undernourished owing to reduced dietary intake, malabsorption and an increased metabolic rate. There is hepatomegaly which may be tender and there may be peritonism. There may be both tricuspid and pulmonary stenosis and/or regurgitation and signs of right heart failure.

Discussion

Primary gastrointestinal carcinoid tumours occur in areas of the embryological foregut (thyroid, bronchus, stomach, common bile duct and pancreas), mid-gut and hind-gut. The most common site is the terminal ileum. Tumours of the bronchus and appendix rarely metastasize. Metabolic symptoms usually occur after there is secondary spread to the liver but in the case of the bronchi, testes or ovaries, symptoms sometimes occur without secondary spread.

A classic symptom is flushing and some patients have a chronically reddened skin with a cyanotic facial hue and widespread telangiectasia. Diarrhoea (secretory) is common, profuse and often associated with abdominal pain, nausea and vomiting. Right hypochondrial pain occurs as a result of hepatomegaly and is severe when the metastases become hypoxic. Peptic ulcer disease is more common in these patients. Involvement of the endocardium of the right heart can cause tricuspid and pulmonary valve lesions and right heart failure. Rarely, carcinoid tumours can synthesize ACTH and be associated with parathyroid adenomas and gastrinomas.

The secretion of 5-hydroxytryptamine (serotonin) and bradykinin by carcinoid tumours causes the symptoms. The diagnosis is confirmed by raised levels of 5-hydroxy indole acetic acid (a metabolite of serotonin) in a 24-hour urine collection. Histologically the cells of a carcinoid tumour reduce silver salts (argentaffin-positive).

Treatment consists of a low serotonin diet (avoid bananas, pineapples and walnuts), serotonin antagonists (cyproheptadine), phenothiazines (control flushing by blocking kallikrein release) and cytotoxic drugs, but the tumours are relatively insensitive to these. Surgery may be curative in some cases and hepatic metastases can be selectively embolized via a hepatic artery catheter, but these procedures are not without risk.

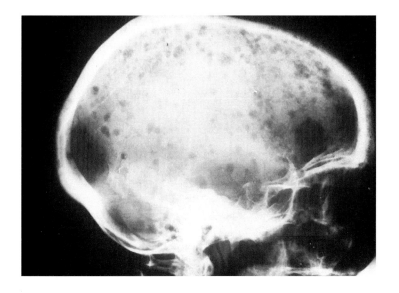

Questions

This 55-year old man complained of backache, polydipsia and polyuria. His wife complained that his snoring had recently kept her awake at night.

(a) What abnormalities can be seen on his skull X-ray?

(b) What is the diagnosis?

(c) What is the cause of his polyuria and polydipsia?

(d) Why had he recently started snoring?

Answers

(a)   Multiple lytic ('punched out') lesions are present
(b)   Multiple myeloma.
(c)   Hypercalcaemia.
(d)   Due to macroglossia caused by secondary amyloidosis.

Short case

There may be evidence of infection (due to immunodeficiency), e.g. pneumonia. There is an abnormal bleeding tendency (bruises, petechial haemorrhages) and anaemia (pallor, tachycardia). There may be bone tenderness and secondary vertebral collapse may produce a paraplegia. Secondary amyloidosis can cause macroglossia and carpal tunnel syndrome as well as a peripheral neuropathy. An associated hyperviscosity syndrome can cause confusion, visual disturbance (due to a retinal vein thrombosis), peripheral neuropathy and heart failure.

If shown the skull X-ray the differential diagnosis of lytic lesions includes myeloma, secondary bone metastases and hyperparathyroidism.

Discussion

Multiple myeloma is a neoplastic monoclonal proliferation of plasma cells characterized by lytic bone lesions, plasma cell accumulation in the bone marrow (>10% but usually >30%) and the presence of a mono-clonal paraprotein in serum and urine (Bence-Jones protein, light chains). The serum paraprotein is IgG in two-thirds of cases, and IgA in one third; IgM or IgD and mixed cases are rare. There is usually a normochromic/normocytic or macrocytic anaemia and there may be rouleaux formation, neutropenia and thrombocytopenia. Other features include plasma cells in the blood (15% of cases), leuco-erythroblastic changes, high erythrocyte sedimentation rate (ESR), hypercalcaemia (45% of cases), uraemia (20% of cases) (due to heavy Bence-Jones pro-teinuria, hypercalcaemia, uric acid, amyloid and pyelonephritis) and a low serum albumin. Clinical features consist of:

● Bone pain/pathological fracture.
● Anaemia, abnormal bleeding tendency.
● Recurrent infection.
● Renal failure.
● Hypercalcaemia (polyuria and polydipsia).
● Amyloidosis (carpal tunnel syndrome, macroglossia, peripheral neuropathy).
● Hyperviscosity syndrome (confusion, peripheral neuropathy, visual field defects, heart failure).

Melphalan or cyclophosphamide with or without prednisolone are the drugs of choice in treatment. Allopurinol is given to prevent attacks of gout and urate nephropathy. Bad prognostic features are: urea >14 mmol/l, serum albumin <30 g/l, Bence-Jones proteinuria >200 mg/dl and haemoglobin < 8 g/dl. The median survival is 2 years with a 20% 4-year survival.

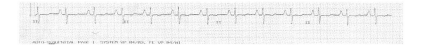

Questions

This is a rhythm strip of a 25-year-old woman with primary pulmonary hypertension.

(a) What is the abnormality on the ECG?

(b) What is the cause of this?

(c) What other features will be on the 12-lead ECG?

(d) Name two other conditions that may cause this ECG appearance.

Answers

(a) A large P wave (P pulmonale, >2.5 mm in height).
(b) Right atrial hypertrophy.
(c) Right ventricular hypertrophy/strain pattern (large R waves in V1–V3, ST depression in V1–V3, right bundle branch block).
(d) These are the causes of pulmonary hypertension:
  (i) Chronic bronchitis.
  (ii) Left heart disease (mitral stenosis, left ventricular failure).
  (iii) Left-to-right shunts (atrial septal defect (ASD), Ventricular septal defect (VSD), Patent Ductus Arteriosus (PDA)).
  (iv) Pulmonary emboli.
  (v) Other pulmonary diseases (rare) – pulmonary fibrosis, asthma, bronchiectasis, emphysema, sarcoidosis.

Short Case

Signs of pulmonary hypertension include malar flush, a large *a* wave in the jugular venous pressure (JVP) caused by atrial contraction and giant *v* waves if there is tricuspid regurgitation, left parasternal heave (caused by right ventricular hypertrophy or from a large pulmonary artery), loud pulmonary second sound, pulmonary early systolic ejection click, right ventricular fourth heart sound, pansystolic murmur of functional tricuspid regurgitation and an early diastolic murmur of functional pulmonary regurgitation (Graham-Steell murmur).

Discussion

The underlying cause of primary pulmonary hypertension is obscure but it occurs in young females and there is often a family history. The prognosis is poor. Vasodilators such as calcium antagonists and prostaglandins have been used with poor results. Most require heart/lung transplantation for cure.

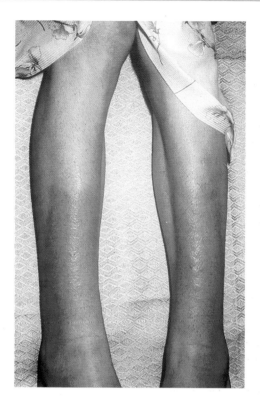

Questions

This woman complained of diarrhoea and weight loss.

(a) What is the skin lesion?

(b) What is the cause of her symptoms?

Answers

(a) Pretibial myxoedema.
(b) Hyperthyroidism.

Short case

Look for signs of thyrotoxicosis: tachycardia (atrial fibrillation), palmar erythema, warm moist hands, exophthalmos, lid retraction, goitre (listen for bruit) or a scar from a previous thyroidectomy.

Discussion

In pretibial myxoedema the lesions are elevated and purple/red in colour. The skin is shiny with well defined margins and an orange peel appearance. The area is tender and itchy. The lesions may also occur in other parts of the body such as the face and are due to infiltration of mucopolysaccharide and hyaluronic acid. It occurs in 5% of patients with Graves' disease. It usually occurs after the onset of treatment (4–30 months). It can be treated with potent steroid ointments under polythene occlusion each night.

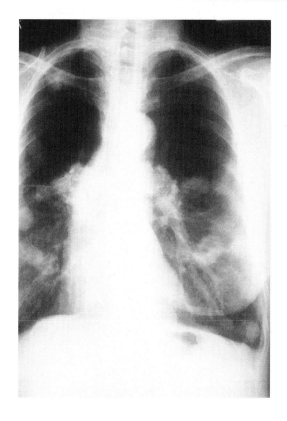

Questions

(a) What is the diagnosis on this chest X-ray?

(b) Name three possible causes.

Answers

(a) Multiple pulmonary metastases. There are large round lesions ('Cannonball') most likely as a result of blood borne spread.

(b) Primary tumours that metastasize to lung include bronchial, renal, breast, thyroid, adrenal, seminomas and sarcomas.

Short Case

Multiple pulmonary metastases are often asymptomatic and are found on routine chest X-ray. The patient often has signs of cancer cachexia. Other symptoms and signs may be related to the primary tumour.

Discussion

If pulmonary metastases are secondary to a unilateral adenocarcinoma of the kidney (5% are bilateral) then nephrectomy may result in spontaneous regression of the metastases.

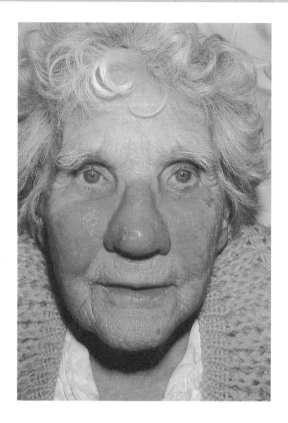

Questions

This 80-year-old woman had a fever.

(a) What is the diagnosis?

(b) What is the cause?

(c) What is the treatment?

Answers

(a)   Erysipelas. Classical 'butterfly' distribution of the rash.
(b)   Group A streptococcal infection.
(c)   Intravenous benzylpenicillin.

Short case

There is a red, inflamed raised area with margins. The leg is another common site of this condition. If severe, there is facial oedema and periorbital puffiness and one or both eyes may be closed. Vesicles and bullae containing clear fluid may appear which rupture and become crusted. The patient is toxic: pyrexial, tachycardia, dehydrated. It is distinguished from maxillary zoster by the unilateral distribution of the rash and vesicular eruption on the palate in the latter condition.

Discussion

Erysipelas lesions may be seen to have arisen from adjacent infected wounds. It is more common in the elderly. The source of the group A streptococci is human and is often carried in the patient's nose. The organism may be isolated not only from the lesion but also from the patient's nose or throat. The disease tends to recur in some patients. It is almost always sensitive to penicillin. Intravenous fluids and intravenous penicillin must be given in the early stages.

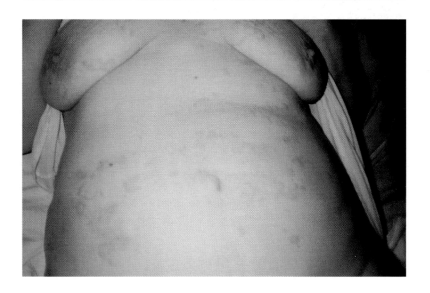

Questions

This woman had suffered a myocardial infarction and had been commenced on aspirin 150 mg daily.

(a) What is the diagnosis?

(b) What is the probable cause in this case?

(c) Name two other possible causes of this condition.

(d) What is the treatment?

Answers

(a) Urticaria.
(b) Aspirin.
(c) In 50% of cases a cause is not found. Recognized causes include:
  (i) Drugs – penicillin, salicylates, isoniazid, codeine.
  (ii) Foods – shellfish, strawberries, pork, eggs.
  (iii) Parasites – fleas, lice, intestinal worms, scabies
  (iv) Inhalants – house dust, feathers.
  (v) Physical – heat, cold, pressure.
  (vi) Cancers – Hodgkins disease, leukaemia, melanoma, mycosis fungoides.
(d) Remove the cause (in this case aspirin), oral antihistamines and topical calamine.

Short Case

This is unlikely to be seen as a short case as it is usually transient (less than 48 hours). There are visible irregular wheals with areas of coalescence. The surface may be smooth, vesicular or bullous and they are red although central blanching may occur. Any area of the skin may be involved and the mucous membranes are often involved, particularly the larynx. The rash is intensely itchy.

Discussion

Urticaria is an acute, chronic or recurrent disorder. Often (50% of cases) no cause is found. Other causes are listed above, the most common being a type I allergic reaction. The agents causing the skin lesions are histamine, serotonin and kinins which are released in response to the antigen/stimulus. Urticaria is more common in women than men and more common between the ages of 30 and 40 years but can occur at any age.

Histologically there is vasodilatation with an infiltrate of white cells. Eosinophilia is common and a total lymphocyte count may be reduced in chronic urticaria.

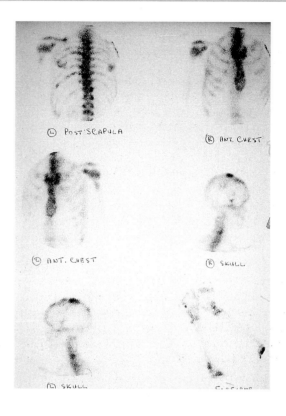

(L) POST SCAPULA   (R) ANT. CHEST

(L) ANT. CHEST   (R) SKULL

(L) SKULL

Questions

(a) What is this investigation?

(b) What does it show?

(c) Name two possible causes.

Answers

(a) An isotope bone scan (technetium-99 methylene diphosphonate is the label in this case).

(b) Multiple bony metastases. Increased areas of uptake can be seen, e.g. skull, ribs.

(c) Tumours that metastasize to the bone include bronchial, breast, thyroid, prostate and sarcomas.

Short Case

Bone metastases may be asymptomatic. There may be areas of tenderness or evidence of a pathological fracture (plaster of Paris, internal fixation is usually required) in a patient with a bronchial carcinoma, as well as clubbing, Horner's syndrome and chest signs in the lung apex.

Discussion

Bone scans are performed by using intravenous phosphate complexes which are labelled with technetium-99. They are more accurate in detecting bone secondaries than plain X-rays; however, it is important to note that positive bone scans can be found in some benign lesions of bone, e.g. Paget's disease, fracture, osteoarthritis, rheumatoid arthritis and inflammatory bone lesions. It is therefore vital to interpret scans in relation to a recent plain X-ray.

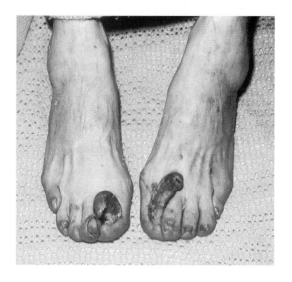

Question

What is the diagnosis?

Answer

Onychogryphosis.

Discussion

The nails are curved and greatly thickened. It may be due to trauma (badly fitting shoes). It is often due to self-neglect and is more common in the elderly and in vagrants. Chiropody is required. In severe cases (as shown) the nails need to be surgically removed.

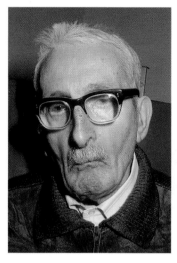 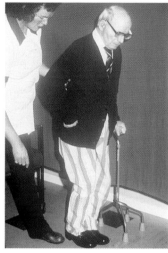

Questions

These two men have the same disease.

(a) What is the diagnosis?

(b) Name two symptoms they may have.

(c) Name two drugs used in the treatment of this condition.

Answers

(a)   *Parkinson's disease. Note the typical 'mask-like' (expressionless) face with greasy skin and a typical posture with flexion of all joints (usually except interphalangeal joints).

(b)   Tremor, slowness, small handwriting (micrographia), increased salivation, dysphagia, constipation, depression and poor memory (dementia is associated).

(c)   Levodopa, usually in combination with a dopa-decarboxylase inhibitor, e.g. Madopar (benserazide), Sinemet (carbidopa) to reduce the extracerebral side-effects of levodopa such as anorexia, nausea or vomiting; selegiline (a monoamine-oxidase inhibitor type B which increases the level of endogenous dopamine by preventing its breakdown), amantadine (an antiviral drug); bromocriptine, lysuride, pergolide and apomorphine are all dopamine receptor agonists. Entacapone is used in combination with Madopar for 'end of dose' motor fluctuations. Anticholinergic drugs such as Benzhexol are less commonly used, especially in the elderly, owing to their adverse side-effects, particularly confusion.

Short Case

The patient is slow and has a resting tremor ('pill rolling') which is decreased by intention. The face is expressionless and unblinking. There is bradykinesia and cog-wheel rigidity (best demonstrated at the wrist and elbow). There is a shuffling gait and balance is poor. Speech may be slow and monotonous and there will be a positive glabella tap (an unreliable sign). The features are usually asymmetrical.

Discussion

Parkinson's disease is more common in men (3:1). It has a prevalence of 1 in 1000 in the UK and is more common in the elderly (1 in 200 of those aged over 70 years). It is characterized by a triad of tremor, rigidity and bradykinesia. It is a progressive neurodegenerative condition. The effects of levodopa diminish after several years and patients experience peak dose toxicity (orofacial dyskinesia and athetoid movements of the trunk and limbs). Refractory hypokinesia with abrupt changes occurs ('on-off' phenomenon). Drugs are therefore being used in combination earlier in the disease process. Other treatments (surgical) are still under trial for this disease. Other causes of the parkinsonian syndrome include:

- Drugs, e.g. phenothiazines, prochlorperazine.
- Brain damage – trauma, anoxia, carbon monoxide and manganese poisoning.
- Post-encephalitis (rare, encephalitis lethargica, panepidemic 1916–1928).

- Cerebral tumours.
- Neurosyphilis.

There are other conditions that have parkinsonian features, e.g. normal pressure hydrocephalus (urinary incontinence, gait apraxia, dementia), Steele-Richardson syndrome (supranuclear gaze palsy, pyramidal signs, dementia, frontal lobe syndrome), Shy-Drager syndrome (idiopathic orthostatic hypotension, cerebellar and pyramidal signs, impotence, incontinence, peripheral neuropathy), Alzheimer's disease, Wilson's disease (Kayser-Fleischer rings, dysarthria, chorea, hepatic cirrhosis, dementia), hypoparathyroidism (basal ganglia calcification) and Jakob-Creutzfeldt disease (slow virus, encephalopathy, dementia, myoclonus, aphasia, cerebellar ataxia, spasticity and cortical blindness).

*J. Parkinson (1755–1824). English physician.

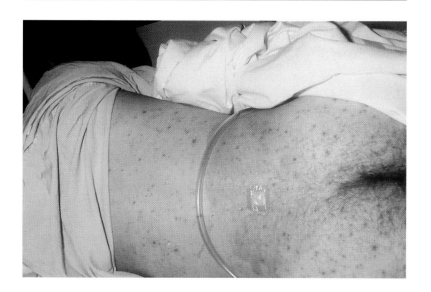

Questions

(a) Name the physical sign in this photograph.

(b) What is the diagnosis?

(c) Name two complications of this condition.

(d) What is the treatment?

CASE 34

Answers

(a) There is a widespread purpuric rash. Also note elastoplast from the lumbar puncture and the urinary catheter to monitor urine output accurately (patient is often confused/drowsy).

(b) Meningococcal meningitis/septicaemia.

(c) Deafness (5%), IIIrd, IVth, VIth or VIIth cranial nerve palsies (transient), hydrocephalus (uncommon), polyarthritis (does not leave permanent joint damage) and pericarditis.

(d) Intravenous benzylpenicillin in high doses (1200 mg every 4 hours) for 7 days. In fulminating septicaemia intravenous plasma, hydrocortisone and oxygen are needed. Dialysis may be required. Treatment should be commenced if this diagnosis is suspected and should not be delayed for a lumbar puncture.

Short Case

This is unlikely to occur as a short case. The differential diagnosis of a purpuric rash includes:

- Vascular
  - Henoch-Schönlein purpura (rash is characteristically on the extremities and buttocks).
  - Scurvy.
  - von Willebrand's disease.
- Thrombocytopenia
  - Idiopathic.
  - Infective: infectious mononucleosis, hepatitis, rubella.
  - Blood dyscrasia: leukaemia.
  - Drugs: busulphan, azathioprine, gold salts, chloramphenicol.
  - Disseminated intravascular coagulation.

Discussion

The causative organism is *Neisseria meningitidis*, a Gram-negative diplococcus. It can occur at any age but is most common in children aged under 5 years.

The incubation period is 1–3 days. The disease starts abruptly with pyrexia, malaise, headache and vomiting. After 24 hours the patient becomes irritable and progression to confusion, drowsiness, coma and convulsions occurs. The rash occurs in 50% of cases. Signs of meningeal irritation are apparent (neck stiffness, head retraction and Kernig's sign). Waterhouse-Friderichsen syndrome is a rapidly fatal presentation with septic shock and disseminated intravascular coagulation when adrenal haemorrhage occurs.

The organism can be isolated in the blood and cerebrospinal fluid

(CSF). Treatment should not be delayed for samples to be taken. CSF is purulent (milky white) with a high white cell count (>500 cells), a raised protein (>2 g/l) and a low/absent sugar concentration. If antibiotics were given before the lumbar puncture then the CSF may be sterile in which case the diagnosis can be confirmed by demonstration of bacterial antigen in the CSF by counter immunophoresis.

The overall mortality is 5–10%. Fulminating septicaemia and unconsciousness on presentation have a higher mortality. Close contacts are given a short course of rifampicin or minocycline to prevent infection.

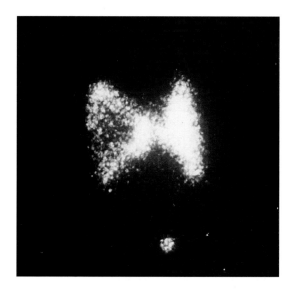

Questions

This 30-year-old woman had evidence of a cervical lymphadenopathy.

(a) What is this investigation?

(b) What does it show?

(c) What is the most likely cause?

(d) What is the treatment?

CASE 35

Answers

(a)   A radioisotope (Iodine–125 is used) scan of the thyroid gland.
(b)   A 'cold nodule' (non-functioning) in the right lobe of the thyroid gland.
(c)   In view of the age and cervical lymphadenopathy a papillary cell carcinoma is most probable.
(d)   All single nodules should be excised to confirm the diagnosis. Treatment of papillary cell carcinoma includes total thyroidectomy and lifelong thyroxine. These tumours are TSH dependent.

Short Case

There is a solitary nodule in the thyroid gland which may be enlarged. The differential diagnosis is thyroid carcinoma, benign adenoma, cyst or haematoma. Other features depend on the histological type of the carcinoma. Papillary carcinomas have an incomplete capsule and metastasize to cervical lymph nodes. Follicular cell tumours produce functioning secondaries (tachycardia, fine tremor, palmar erythema, sweating). Anaplastic tumours usually cause a hard, enlarged gland and are highly malignant, being more common in the elderly. Medullary cell tumours may be associated with mucosal neuromas, marfanoid habitus, proximal myopathy and skin pigmentation (MEA type IIB, see below), and may secrete ACTH.

Discussion

Thyroid carcinomas are rare. They are found most commonly in women aged 45–65 years. Ionising radiation in childhood is a pre-disposing factor. There are four types:

1. **Papillary**. This is the most common and occurs in the relatively young. It is TSH dependent and regresses with thyroxine. A total thyroidectomy should be performed.
2. **Follicular**. Often this produces functioning secondaries that are sensitive to radioiodine. A total thyroidectomy should be performed.
3. **Anaplastic.** This has a poor prognosis and occurs mainly in the elderly. Surgical removal should not be attempted but this is sometimes necessary to relieve pressure symptoms. Radioiodine is not effective and treatment is with external radiation.
4. **Medullary.** This is rare. It may secret calcitonin, ACTH, serotonin or prostaglandins. It carries a good prognosis. It is associated with MEA type IIA (Sipple's syndrome) (medullary cell carcinoma of the thyroid, phaeochromocytoma, parathyroid hyperplasia). It is sometimes associated with mucosal neuromas, marfenoid habitus, skin pigmentation, proximal myopathy and intestinal abnormalities (megacolon and ganglioneuroma). This is MEA type IIB, which is also autosomal

dominant. Relatives of patients with medullary cell carcinoma should be screened for this and other endocrine neoplasia.

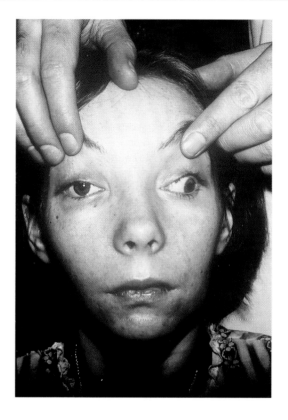

Questions

This young girl feels better in the morning.

(a) Name two physical signs.

(b) Name two symptoms she may have.

(c) What is the diagnosis?

(d) Name three other diseases that may be associated with this condition.

(e) Name one drug used in the treatment of this condition.

Answers

(a) Strabismus, bilateral ptosis and lack of expression caused by facial muscle weakness.

(b) Diplopia, proximal muscle weakness (fatiguability), dysphagia, weakness of speech, breathlessness (this is a sinister sign).

(c) Myasthenia gravis.

(d) Autoimmune diseases, e.g. thyrotoxicosis, hypothyroidism, rheumatoid arthritis, SLE, diabetes mellitus, pernicious anaemia, polymyositis, pemphigus and sarcoidosis.

(e) Long-acting anticholinesterase, e.g. neostigmine or pyridostigmine. Thymectomy improves 70% of cases. Steroids and immunosuppressants may be useful. Plasmapheresis has been used in severe cases.

Short Case

The patient will have ptosis (may be bilateral) and a variable strabismus which is made worse after making the patient move the muscles involved. Facial muscles are weak. There is a proximal myopathy (upper limbs more than lower limbs). There may be a sternotomy scar due to a thymectomy. There may be evidence of associated disease, e.g. rheumatoid hands, butterfly rash in SLE. The differential diagnosis is:

- Other causes of ptosis – IIIrd cranial nerve lesion, Horner's syndrome, dystrophia myotonica, congenital facio-scapulo-humeral dystrophy, tabo-paresis.
- Familial hypokalaemic paralysis.
- *Eaton-Lambert syndrome. This is associated with oat cell carcinoma of the bronchus. Proximal muscle weakness and wasting are prevalent and the power is often increased by exercise initially. Facial muscles are less often involved. There is no response to Edrophonium but weakness is improved by guanidine hydrochloride.

Discussion

Myasthenia gravis is a rare disorder of muscle weakness caused by failure of neuromuscular transmission and is more common in women (2:1). The number of postsynaptic acetylcholine receptors are reduced and anti-acetylcholine receptor antibodies are present in the serum in 90% of cases. Thymomas occur in 10–20% of cases (mainly males) and are associated with a worse prognosis.

The diagnosis is confirmed by the Tensilon test (edrophonium 10 mg i.v. reduces weakness of the affected muscles for about 3 minutes). There should be a CT scan of the anterior mediastinum to exclude a thymoma. Long-term treatment is described above. A myasthenic crisis may be precipitated by exertion, infection, emotion or drugs (quinine, quinidine, gentamycin, neomycin, procainamide). Overtreatment results in a cholinergic crisis with symptoms of confusion, vomiting, abdominal pain, sweating and pallor which is sometimes difficult to differentiate from a myasthenic crisis and therefore requires drug withdrawal and assisted ventilation for a short period.

The prognosis is variable and the disease may never progress beyond an ophthalmoplegia or death may occur rapidly due to involvement of respiratory muscles. Thymomas are associated with a worse prognosis.

*L.M. Eaton (1905–1958). American neurologist.

*E.H. Lambert. American neurophysiologist.

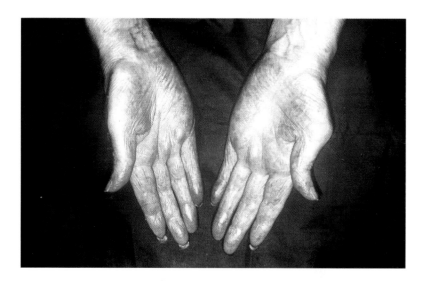

Questions

These are the hands of a 58-year-old woman with xanthelasma who presented with a haematemesis.

(a) What is the physical sign shown?

(b) What is the diagnosis?

(c) Name three other signs that may be present in her hands.

(d) What is the likely cause of her haematemesis?

Answers

(a) Palmar erythema ('liver palms').
(b) Primary biliary cirrhosis.
(c) Other hand signs of chronic liver disease include: finger clubbing, spider naevi, leuconychia, Dupuytren's contracture, jaundice, pallor, pigmentation and purpura.
(d) Oesophageal varices.

Short Case

The patient will be jaundiced with skin pigmentation and scratch marks (caused by pruritus). Xanthomas are present (over site of trauma). Other signs of chronic liver disease are described above. There will be hepatosplenomegaly.

Discussion

Primary biliary cirrhosis mainly affects women (90% of cases). It is associated with other immunological disorders: rheumatoid arthritis, Hashimoto's thyroiditis, dermatomyositis, Crest syndrome and Sjögren's syndrome and coeliac disease. Serum anti-mitochondrial antibodies are present in 95%, smooth muscle antibodies in 50% and anti-nuclear factor in 20% of cases. The alkaline phosphatase and bilirubin levels are raised as a result of cholestatic jaundice.

Treatment is with cholestyramine for pruritus and supplements of fat soluble vitamins, calcium and phosphate. Ursodeoxycholic acid improves liver function tests but has no effect on survival. Penicillamine may improve survival in advanced disease. Death from hepatocellular failure with or without bleeding occurs within 5–10 years.

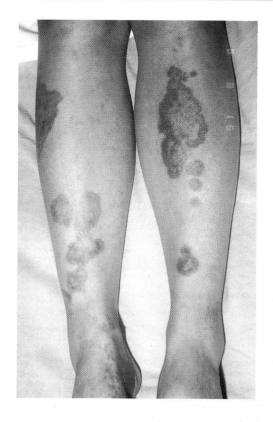

Questions

(a) What is the diagnosis?

(b) What is the treatment?

Answers

(a)   Necrobiosis lipoidica diabeticorum.

(b)   If diabetes is present (may occur in pre-diabetic state), good diabetic control may improve its appearance. Steroids (topical or local injections) may help. Severe cases may be treated by excision and skin grafting.

Short Case

Look for other skin lesions associated with diabetes:

- Infections.
- Vitiligo.
- Xanthelasma.
- Pseudoxanthoma nigricans.
- Peripheral anhydrosis (due to autonomic neuropathy).

Fundoscopy may reveal a retinopathy.

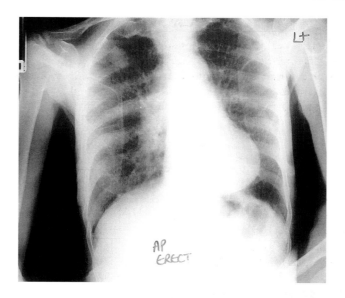

Questions

This 70-year-old man presented with a severe nose bleed. Results of his blood tests revealed: Hb 8.1 g/dl, white cell count 2.1 x 10⁹/l, platelets 27 x 10⁹/l, calcium 2.63 mmol/l, albumin 20 g/l.

(a) Describe the abnormalities on his chest X-ray.

(b) What is the diagnosis?

(c) Name two possible causes of this condition.

(d) What is the probable cause of his pancytopenia?

(e) What is his corrected calcium level and list two causes for this.

Answers

(a) There is a rounded/oval lesion in the right upper zone and an enlarged right hilum.

(b) Bronchial carcinoma in the right apex with secondary spread to the right hilum or vice versa.

(c) Cigarette smoking or exposure to asbestos, chromium, arsenic or radioactive materials.

(d) Bone marrow failure as a result of tumour infiltration (common with small cell carcinomas).

(e) Corrected calcium level is 3.03 mmol/l ((40–20) $\times$ 0.02 = 0.4 + 2.63 = 3.03 mmol/l, correct calcium to an albumin level of 40 g/l). The reason for the hypercalcaemia may be due to parathormone-related protein secretion by the bronchial carcinoma (squamous cell tumour) or bony metastases.

Short Case

Any of the following may be present on physical examination; finger clubbing, tar staining of the fingers, Horner's syndrome, cervical lymph nodes, hoarse voice (caused by involvement of the recurrent laryngeal nerve), dermatomyositis, acanthosis nigricans, atrial fibrillation and pericarditis (caused by local invasion), superior vena caval obstruction (see case 14), cerebellar syndrome, peripheral neuropathy, proximal myopathy, myasthenic syndrome (Eaton-Lambert syndrome).

Discussion

Bronchial carcinoma is more common in men although the incidence in women is increasing because of increased cigarette smoking. About 40% are squamous, 25% oat cell, 20% large cell, and 15% are adenocarcinomas. Alveolar cell carcinoma is rare.

Surgery offers the only cure but only 10–20% of cases are suitable at presentation. Metastases are present in 60% at presentation. Radiotherapy offers symptomatic relief from pain and haemoptysis. Chemotherapy has been shown to improve survival in small cell carcinoma.

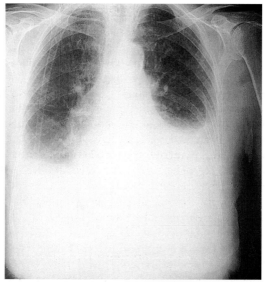

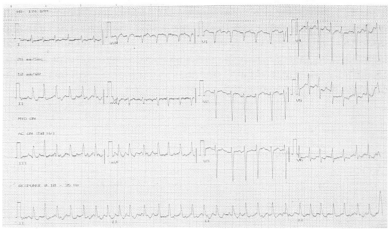

Questions

The chest X-ray and ECG belong to the same patient.

(a) What does the chest X-ray show?

(b) What abnormalities are apparent on the ECG?

(c) Name three causes of the ECG appearance.

CASE 40

Answers

(a) There are bilateral pleural effusions (left more than the right), upper lobe diversion and interstitial oedema. The diagnosis is pulmonary oedema resulting from left ventricular failure.

(b) Atrial fibrillation with a ventricular rate of about 150 per minute. There is inferolateral ischaemia.

(c) Causes of atrial fibrillation include: ischaemic heart disease, thyrotoxicosis, mitral valve disease, pulmonary embolism, carcinoma of bronchus, cardiomyopathy, hypertension, atrial septal defect, constrictive pericarditis, atrial myxoma and idiopathic.

Short Case

The patient will be dyspnoeic and may be centrally cyanosed. The pulse is irregularly irregular and the JVP may be raised (*a* waves will be absent). There may be murmurs of mitral and triscupid valve regurgitation as a result of cardiac dilatation but these may be difficult to hear because of the tachycardia. Other murmurs may be present that have precipitated left ventricular failure, e.g. atrial septal defect (pulmonary systolic ejection murmur caused by increased flow, right ventricular heave, tricuspid diastolic flow murmur). There will be clinical signs of bilateral pleural effusions (decreased expansion of the chest, dullness to percussion, absent or bronchial breath sounds) and crackles will be audible owing to interstitial oedema.

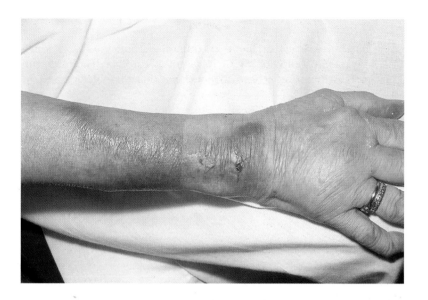

Questions

This is the arm of the woman whose chest X-ray and ECG can be seen in case 40.

(a) What does it show?

(b) Name two possible causes of this appearance.

Answers

(a) There is extensive erythema surrounding a punctured area which is most probably due to an intravenous cannula. These appearances are consistent with a superficial thrombophlebitis and/or overlying cellulitis.

(b) Superficial thrombophlebitis and cellulitis may have been caused by infection introduced by the intravenous cannula. Superficial thrombophlebitis can also be caused by intravenous amiodarone and potassium solutions. These are irritant to the veins. Parenteral amiodarone should be given through large vessels, i.e. through a subclavian line. Intravenous potassium should not be given in concentrations >20 mmol in 500 ml of solution.

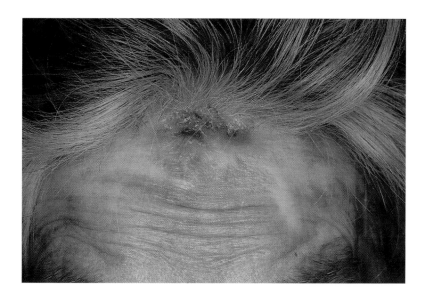

Questions

This woman is demented. This skin lesion always responded to hospitalization and reappeared after discharge.

(a) What is the diagnosis?

(b) What is the treatment?

Answers

(a) Dermatitis artefacta. This refers to a skin lesion that is self-inflicted with no obvious underlying cause, e.g. pruritus. The unusual position of the skin lesion and chronic fibrotic changes surrounding it suggest it may be self-inflicted. It healed in hospital as nursing staff discouraged this lady from picking her scalp area.

(b) Determine the underlying cause, e.g. malingerers, psychosis, and treat this. Lesions should be treated with occlusive dressings and it may be necessary to observe as an inpatient.

Short Case (see Appendix, Figure 10)

The skin lesion will have a curious shape and notably will resemble no other disorder. The lesions will often possess angles and edges. The patient usually denies how the lesion developed. The severity of the lesion depends on the agent used, which include cigarettes, sand paper, matches, knives or carbolic acid. It is unlikely that an examiner will expect a psychiatric history to be taken as this is time consuming and this is usually a 'spot' diagnosis.

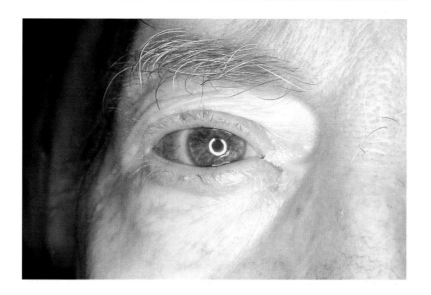

Questions

This man had a painful right eye 6 months previously.

(a) What is the physical sign?

(b) What was the cause of his red eye?

(c) Name two diseases associated with this condition.

Answers

(a) Scleromalacia (translucency of the sclera).

(b) Scleritis. When the sclera heals it becomes transluscent and the blue/black underlying choroid can be seen. The translucent sclera is not thinned despite the appearance. Complications of scleritis include glaucoma and cataracts.

(c) (i) Rheumatoid arthritis – other occular disease associated with this includes scleromalacia perforans when necrotizing scleritis may lead to perforation of the sclera and keratoconjunctivitis sicca. (Cataracts occur as a result of Chloroquine and steroids.)

(ii) Ulcerative colitis.

(iii) Crohn's disease.

Short Case

The patient may have clinical signs of rheumatoid disease which can be noted quickly: arthropathy (look at the hands), anaemia (pallor) and leg ulcer (vasculitis). Specifically, examination of the chest and cardiovascular system may reveal features related to rheumatoid disease (pleural effusion, pulmonary fibrosis, pericarditis, mitral and/or aortic valve regurgitation).

Discussion

Scleritis is a deep inflammation of the sclera and is distinguishable from the more superficial, innocuous episcleritis. It occurs in rheumatoid disease in association with vasculitis and other systemic complications. The symptoms vary from minimal discomfort to excruciating pain.

Treatment of scleritis is with local steroid drops and anti-inflammatory drugs in the first instance. Sometimes systemic steroids are required for severe cases.

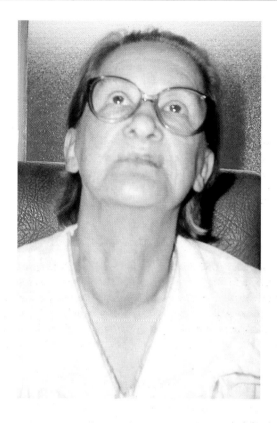

Questions

This woman complained of palpitations.

(a) What abnormality can be seen in this photograph?

(b) What is the diagnosis?

(c) What is the cause of her palpitations?

(d) Name two other symptoms she may have.

(e) What is the treatment?

CASE 44

Answers

(a) A goitre (probably multinodular).

(b) Thyrotoxicosis.

(c) Sinus tachycardia or atrial fibrillation (caused by excess thyroxine potentiating the action of catecholamines).

(d) Tremor, excessive sweating, heat intolerance, weight loss, diarrhoea, breathlessness, tiredness and increased appetite.

(e) Anti-thyroid drug (carbimazole) initially until radioactive iodine is administered. Radioactive iodine is now used for most cases. Propranolol is useful for cardiac symptoms and tremor. Surgery is reserved for failure of medical management, relief of pressure effect, such as dysphagia and cosmetic purposes.

Short Case. (see Appendix, Figure 11)

The patient with thyrotoxicosis is usually female and has a goitre (multinodular in the elderly and smooth and diffuse in the young). Examine the patient from in front with her in the sitting position. Observe the neck closely asking the patient to swallow (a drink of water may be needed). Then examine from behind the patient by gentle palpation with fingers feeling each lobe of the thyroid and ask the patient to swallow again. Listen for a bruit over the goitre which is due to increased blood flow through it.

Other signs include fine tremor (made more obvious by balancing a sheet of paper on the patient's outstretched hands), palmar erythema, sweating palms, acropachy (finger clubbing), onycholysis (*Plummer's nails, typically found bilaterally on the fourth finger), sinus tachycardia/atrial fibrillation/bounding pulse, eye signs (exophthalmos, lid retraction, lid lag, chemosis), proximal muscle weakness (thyrotoxic myopathy), diffuse alopecia, hyper-reflexia and kyphosis secondary to thyrotoxic osteoporosis.

Discussion

The majority of cases of hyperthyroidism are due to a diffuse toxic goitre (Graves' disease) and a toxic nodular goitre. Thyrotoxicosis is more common in women (5:1). Graves' disease is an autoimmune disease and is associated with HLA-B8 and HLA-DR3. There are stimulating antibodies against the TSH receptor site. Rarer causes of the thyrotoxicosis include self-administered thyroxine, carcinoma of the thyroid, Hashimoto's thyroiditis (transient) and a TSH-producing pituitary tumour.

There are some important clinical differences between Graves' disease and a toxic nodular goitre:

Graves' disease	Toxic nodular goitre
Younger	Older
Diffuse enlargement of gland	Nodular enlargement
Eye signs common	Eye signs uncommon
Atrial fibrillation uncommon	Atrial fibrillation common
Autoimmune associations common	Autoimmune associations uncommon

Examples of autoimmune diseases associated with Graves' disease include; diabetes mellitus, pernicious anaemia, Addison's disease, vitiligo, chronic active hepatitis, primary biliary cirrhosis, myasthenia gravis, systemic sclerosis and Sjögren's syndrome. It is also associated with temporal arteritis and polymyalgia rheumatica.

Treatment consists of:
- Antithyroid drugs – carbimazole. Treatment is needed for 12–18 months. However, carbimazole is not without complications (leucopenia, arthralgia and rash) and the relapse rate is high (up to 60%). It is therefore now used until radioiodine therapy is administered or if the patient is pregnant.
- Radioiodine – iodine-131 is now more commonly used even in the young. The gland decreases in size after treatment. It is an atraumatic treatment but the incidence of late hypothyroidism is high (15% at 2 years).
- Propranolol – it is useful to control cardiac symptoms and tremor.
- Surgery – this requires preoperative treatment with carbimazole and potassium iodide. Subtotal thyroidectomy is reserved for failure of medical management, large nodular goitres causing pressure symptoms (dysphagia, dyspnoea, stridor) and cosmetic reasons. Complications of surgery include relapse (5%), hypothyroidism (15%), recurrent laryngeal nerve palsy (rare) and hypoparathyroidism (rare).

Atrial fibrillation associated with thyrotoxicosis is digoxin resistant and larger doses are needed. A beta-blocker may be more useful. Cardioversion may be used. Atrial fibrillation associated with thyrotoxicosis is associated with an increased incidence of thromboembolic phenomenon and therefore anti-coagulation with warfarin should be considered.

Thyrotoxic crisis is rare but dangerous and requires treatment with intravenous dexamethasone, oral carbimazole followed by potassium iodide, beta-blockers, intravenous fluids and oxygen.

Management of thyroid eye disease is considered later in this book.

*H.S Plummer (1874–1936). American physician, Mayo Clinic.

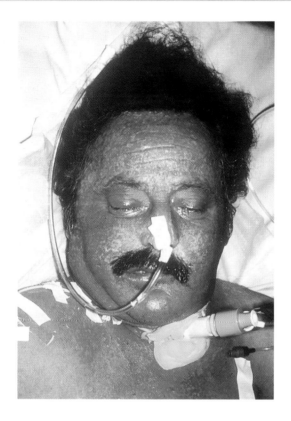

Questions

This man had ingested antifreeze (ethylene glycol) 4 days previously.

(a) Name three abnormalities in this photograph.

(b) Name two initial symptoms (less than 12 hours after ingestion) he may have had.

(c) What is the treatment?

Answers

(a) Tracheostomy for mechanical ventilation, nasogastric tube, left subclavian line and uraemic frost (white crystals of urea on the face). Uraemic frost along with muscular twitching and hiccups are terminal manifestations of renal failure.

(b) Initial symptoms (less than 12 hours after ingestion) are confined to the gastrointestinal and nervous systems, e.g. nausea, vomiting, haematemesis, coma, convulsions. Signs include: a patient who appears intoxicated but without smelling of alcohol, nystagmus, ophthalmoplegia, papilloedema, optic atrophy and myoclonic jerks. After 12–14 hours there is cardiorespiratory involvement and after 3 days renal failure develops (due to acute tubular necrosis).

(c) Early diagnosis reduces mortality. Gastric lavage is needed to prevent further absorption and confirm the diagnosis. Other treatment is supportive to combat shock, hypocalcaemia and metabolic acidosis. Ethyl alcohol is a competitive inhibitor of ethylene glycol and should be used (50 g orally then 10-12 g per hour intravenously) to keep plasma ethanol levels at 1000–2000 mg/l. Dialysis is often required to further eliminate ethylene glycol from the body and to manage the renal complications (acute tubular necrosis).

Discussion

Ethylene glycol (antifreeze) may be ingested acidentally or in a suicide attempt. It is a poor man's substitute for alcohol. The minimal lethal dose is 100 ml. Deaths are uncommon in England and Wales (35 cases in 26 years).

Ethylene glycol is non-toxic but it is metabolized to oxalate and lactic acid, which are toxic. Ingestion should be suspected in the following circumstances;

- An apparently intoxicated patient with no alcohol detectable in blood or breath.
- Coma associated with a metabolic acidosis or hypocalcaemia, hyperkalaemia and renal failure.
- Urine contains calcium oxalate crystals, protein and blood.

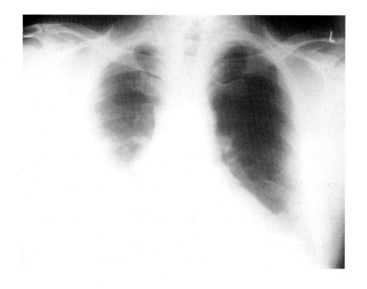

Questions

(a) What is the abnormality on this chest X-ray?

(b) List three possible causes.

Answers

(a)   A right pleural effusion.

(b)   A pleural effusion may be a transudate (increased capillary pressure protein concentration <30 g/l) or an exudate (increased capillary permeability protein concentration >30 g/l). Causes are:

   (i) Transudate – heart failure, hepatic failure, renal failure (effusions are usually bilateral).

   (ii) Exudate – bronchial carcinoma, mesothelioma, pneumonia, tuberculosis, pulmonary embolism, connective tissue diseases (rheumatoid arthritis, SLE) subphrenic abscess, *Meigs' syndrome (associated with ovarian fibroma and ascites).

Short Case

The patient may be breathless at rest. Look for finger clubbing/tar staining (associated with bronchial carcinoma and mesothelioma). The patient may have changes of rheumatoid arthritis in the hands or a 'butterfly' rash associated with SLE. There may be a palpable scalene lymph node (supraclavicular node), associated with respiratory malignancy. The trachea may be deviated with large effusions. There will be decreased expansion on the right with a stony dull percussion note and decreased tactile vocal fremitus. The air entry will be decreased on the right and there may be bronchial breath sounds audible over or above the effusion. Vocal resonance is decreased. These are the signs of a pleural effusion.

*J.V. Meigs (1892–1963). American obstetrician and gynaecologist. Professor of Gynaecology, Harvard and Massachusetts.

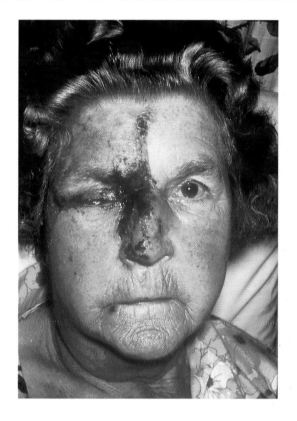

Questions

(a) What is the diagnosis?

(b) Name two possible complications.

(c) What is the treatment?

CASE 47

Answers

(a) Herpes zoster affecting the ophthalmic division of the trigeminal nerve (ophthalmic zoster).

(b) If the nasociliary branch (supplies eye and tip of nose) of the ophthalmic nerve is involved then conjunctivitis, keratitis, iritis and glaucoma may occur. Other complications include long-term scarring, post-herpetic neuralgia and associated depression.

(c) Systemic acyclovir used as early as possible (before lesions have crusted). Strong analgesia. Tricyclic antidepressants (amitriptyline starting at low doses, 10 mg at night) are useful for post-herpetic neuralgia.

Short Case (see Appendix, Figure 12)

The patient has a vesicular rash in an area of skin supplied by the trigeminal nerve (ophthalmic, maxillary or mandibular branch) or another dermatome region. The rash is confined to one half (well demarcated) of the mid-line. The lesions go through several stages: papule, vesicle, pustule, crusting, scarring. The regional lymph nodes are enlarged.

A cranial nerve may be involved. A VIIth cranial nerve palsy with lesions in the external auditory meatus is called *Ramsay Hunt syndrome and is due to zoster of the geniculate ganglion. The VIIIth nerve may be involved (deafness, vertigo) and is common in association with a VIIth nerve palsy.

Peripheral motor nerve lesions, if involved, can result in lower motor neurone signs (paralysis, wasting, fasciculation and decreased reflexes) and a transverse myelitis and cerebellar ataxia can occur.

Discussion

Herpes zoster (shingles) is caused by the varicella-zoster virus. Following chicken-pox the virus persists in the sensory nerves and root ganglia. The activation results in an eruption in the area supplied by the nerve. Non-immune individuals in contact with such patients may develop chicken-pox. Herpes zoster is most common in the elderly but can occur in association with immune deficiency: e.g. leukaemia, Hodgkin's disease, patients on chemotherapy. In the latter, widespread dissemination of the lesions may occur which is associated with a significant mortality.

The condition presents with paraesthesiae and pain in the sensory nerve area a few days before the rash appears. Rarely there is pain but no rash (zoster sine herpete) and diagnosis is confirmed by a raised varicella zoster titre. The eruption is present for 2–3 weeks and it may leave depigmented, anaesthetic areas. Pain may persist (post-herpetic neuralgia, 10% of cases) which is more common in the elderly but less likely if

124

acyclovir is used early. The most common site is a thoracic dermatome followed by ophthalmic zoster.

Other complications include visceral nerve involvement (pain and organ dysfunction), polyneuritis, myelitis and encephalitis, although all of these are rare.

*__J. Ramsey Hunt__ (1874–1937). American neurologist. Professor of Neurology, Columbia University, New York, USA.

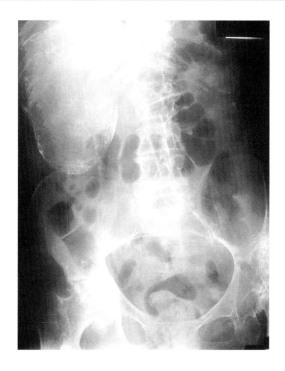

Questions

This Welsh woman was admitted with an acute myocardial infarction.

(a) What abnormality can be seen on her abdominal X-ray?

(b) What is the diagnosis?

(c) What is the cause?

(d) Name two symptoms she may experience as a result of the diagnosis on the abdominal X-ray.

(e) What is the treatment?

Answers

(a) A large, calcified, rounded lesion in the right upper quadrant.

(b) Hydatid cyst of liver.

(c) The tapeworm, *Echinococcus granulosus*. The sheep is an inter-mediate host of this tapeworm and therefore it is significant that she is Welsh as the disease is more common in sheep-farming communities.

(d) Often they are asymptomatic, as in this case, and are noted inci-dentally on a plain X-ray. However, spontaneous rupture may cause sudden pain, fever and allergic reaction.

(e) Surgical removal may be necessary to prevent complications of rupture.

Short Case

The patient would have a palpable mass in the right upper quadrant with-in the liver.

Discussion

Dogs are infected with the tapeworm *Echinococcus granulosus* by eating infected sheep offal. Man becomes infected by close contacts with dogs. The cysts occur mainly in the liver (75% of cases) but can occur in the lung. They may be asymptomatic but can:

- Rupture into the biliary tree, peritoneal cavity, pleural cavity and alimentary canal.
- Become infected.
- Press on bile ducts producing obstructive jaundice.

Cysts can be identified on scans and plain X-rays. Serological tests are positive if the patient has been sensitized to the cyst fluid after leakage. The intradermal *Casoni test is the production of a wheal and flare fol-lowing injection of fresh, sterile hydatid fluid. There may also be an eosinophilia.

An asymptomatic calcified cyst can be left alone as its contents are dead unless it is causing local symptoms from pressure. Other cysts should be removed to prevent complications. Before removal at operation the cyst is injected with formalin or hypertonic saline to kill daughter cysts to prevent spread.

*T. Casoni (1880–1933). Italian physician at the Victor Emanuele III Hospital, Tripoli, Italy.

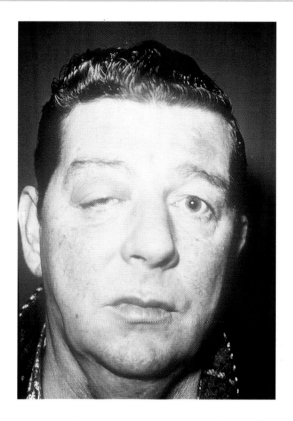

Questions

This 55-year-old man had pain in his right shoulder and complained of numbness over his right forearm.

(a) What physical sign is shown?

(b) What is the diagnosis?

(c) Name two associated features.

(d) What is the cause of the patient's shoulder pain?

(e) Name two other physical signs he may have.

CASE 49

Answers

(a) Right partial ptosis.

(b) Right *Horner's syndrome.

(c) Horner's syndrome consists of miosis, enophthalmos, ptosis, anhy-drosis and vasodilatation of the head and neck on the affected side.

(d) The cause of the pain and the right Horner's syndrome is an apical carcinoma of lung (*Pancoast's syndrome). The apical carcinoma (usually adenocarcinoma) compresses the lower brachial plexus (C8, T1) and the cervical sympathetic nerves.

(e) Other physical signs of a Pancoast's include: wasting of the small muscles of the hand (T1), C7, C8 and T1 sensory loss, finger club-bing, cervical lymph nodes, tracheal deviation and apical chest signs.

Short Case

The patient will have the features of Horner's syndrome as described above. The signs are due to a lesion affecting the sympathetic nervous sys-tem from the sympathetic nucleus, down the brain stem to C8, T1 and T2 leading to the sympathetic chain and then stellate ganglion and carotid sympathetic plexus. Examination of the eyes may be requested and this should be done in sequence as previously described. Other signs may be present depending on the cause of Horner's syndrome:

● Malignant cervical nodes, e.g. lymphoma.
● Neck surgery or trauma (scars?).
● Carotid and aortic aneurysms.
● Syringomyelia (bilateral wasting of the small muscles of the hand, scarred hands, loss of pain and temperature sensation but preserva-tion of touch and proprioception, bulbar palsy, pyramidal signs and nystagmus).
● Idiopathic (most common in females).
● Brain stem vascular disease (lateral medullary syndrome) or *Wallenberg's syndrome   (ipsilateral Vth, IXth, Xth, XIth cranial nerve lesions, cerebellar ataxia, nystagmus and contralateral spinothalamic loss).
● Demyelinating disease.

Discussion

Ptosis can be classified as unilateral or bilateral and its causes are as follows:
● Unilateral – Horner's syndrome, congenital, IIIrd cranial nerve palsy, myasthenia gravis, dystrophia myotonica.

- Bilateral – same as unilateral causes and also tabes dorsalis, occular myopathy (absence of soft tissue in the eyelids, face and neck weakness, ophthalmoplegia), oculopharyngeal muscular dystrophy (ocular myopathy features and dysphagia).

*J.F. Horner (1831–1886) Swiss ophthalmologist. Professor of Ophthalmology, Zurich, Switzerland.

*H.K. Pancoast (1875–1939) American radiologist. Professor of Radiology, University of Pennsylvania, USA.

*A. Wallenberg (1862–1949) German neurologist.

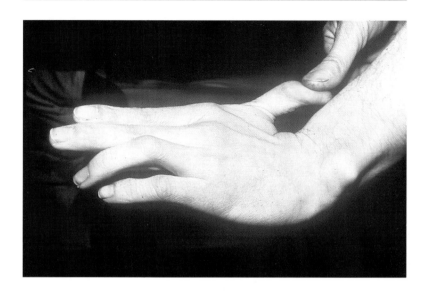

Questions

This patient, a 20-year-old man, had extensive bruising. He had a late systolic murmur.

(a) What physical sign is demonstrated?

(b) What is the cause of his heart murmur?

(c) What is the diagnosis?

(d) Name two other complications of this condition.

Answers

(a)   Hyperextensibility of the first metacarpophalangeal joint.
(b)   Mitral valve prolapse (a 'floppy' mitral valve).
(c)   *Ehlers-Danlos syndrome.
(d)   Poorly healing skin, spontaneous bleeding (usually from the gut), diaphragmatic herniae, scleromalacia, spontaneous pneumothorax, spontaneous rupture of large arteries and dissecting aneurysms.

Short Case

The patient is of normal or short stature (unlike Marfan's syndrome which has some similar clinical features) with thin, pale, hyperextensile skin with prominent veins. There may be bruises and many scars and hyperextensile joints. The patient often has myopia and flat feet.

Discussion

Ehlers-Danlos syndrome is a term applied to a group of conditions in which there is defective collagen giving rise to the above symptoms and signs. There are eight types, which vary in prominence and severity of clinical features and inheritance pattern. Inheritance patterns include dominant, recessive and X-linked.

Symptoms of mitral valve prolapse include chest pain, fatigue, palpitations and dyspnoea. It may be asymptomatic. A floppy mitral valve affects 5–10% of the population. When there is an audible murmur and the diagnosis is confirmed on echocardiogram there is an increased risk of bacterial endocarditis and the patient requires antibiotic prophylaxis for dental procedures, etc. Other congenital cardiac defects may occur with this syndrome, for example atrial septal defects are common.

Other conditions associated with hyperextensile joints include Marfan's syndrome, Turner's syndrome, Noonan's syndrome, Down's syndrome, pseudoxanthoma elasticum and osteogenesis imperfecta.

*E. Ehlers (1863–1937). Danish dermatologist. Professor of Dermatology, Copenhagen.

*H. A. Danlos (1844–1912). French physician and dermatologist.

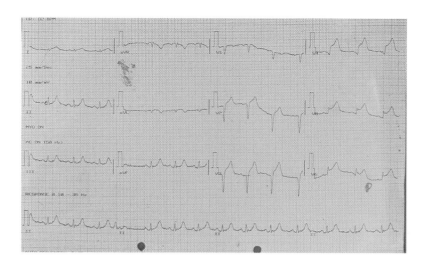

Questions

(a) What is the diagnosis on this ECG?

(b) What is the treatment?

(c) List three possible complications from this disease.

Answers

(a) Acute anterior myocardial infarction. There is ST elevation in V2–V6 and anterior septal Q waves.
(b) Thrombolysis and aspirin unless there are contraindications.
(c) Arrhythmias, left ventricular failure, shock, ventricular septal defect, rupture of chordae causing mitral regurgitation, pericarditis, left ventricular aneurysm and *Dressler's syndrome (pleural effusion, fever, anaemia, high ESR).

Short Case

The patient may be included in the examination a few weeks post-infarction. This may be because there are some significant complications, e.g. atrial fibrillation. A ventricular septal defect may be present (a displaced apex beat, pansystolic murmur left sternal edge, a mid-diastolic murmur may be present if the shunt is large). It may be clinically difficult to distinguish from mitral regurgitation. An echocardiogram would solve the dilemma.

Rarely patients who have had a myocardial infarction can subsequently develop undetected ventricular septal defects and present later with features of *Eisenmenger's syndrome. This is when a left to right shunt is reversed owing to the development of pulmonary hypertension. The clinical features consist of: finger clubbing, central cyanosis, large *a* wave in the JVP and a large *v* wave if tricuspid regurgitation is present, a left parasternal heave, a displaced apex beat, loud second heart sound, fourth heart sound and the murmurs of pulmonary regurgitation and tricuspid regurgitation. This carries with it a poor prognosis and treatment is symptomatic and surgery contraindicated.

A left ventricular aneurysm is another complication which may arise and this results in persistent ST elevation in the ECG. There is also a double impulse on palpation of the apex beat. Complications of a left ventricular aneurysm include ventricular arrhythmia, left ventricular failure, rupture and cardiac tamponade, thromboembolic phenomenon (e.g. stroke), femoral embolus and mesenteric vascular embolus.

*V. Eisenmenger (1864–1932). German physician.

*W. Dressler (1890–1969). American cardiologist.

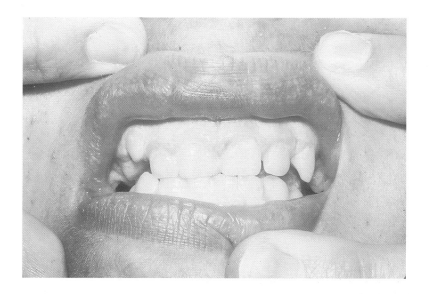

Questions

(a) What is the diagnosis?

(b) Name two diseases that cause this condition.

(c) Name a drug that may cause this.

Answers

(a)   Gum hypertrophy.
(b)   Scurvy, periodontal disease and leukaemia (especially acute myelomonocytic leukaemia).
(c)   Phenytoin and nifedipine.

Short Case

Scurvy (vitamin C deficiency) may still be seen, particularly amongst the elderly who sometimes live on 'toast and tea'. Other physical signs to look for are purpura, often on the thigh just above the knees, perifollicular haemorrhages, pigmentation, broken hairs on the limbs, bleeding gums and haemarthroses.

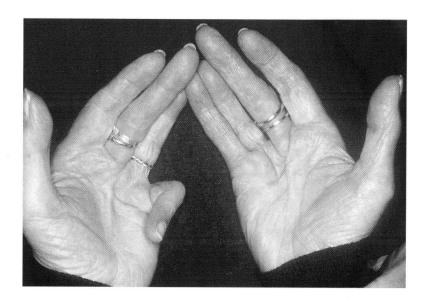

Questions

(a) What is the diagnosis?

(b) Name two possible causes.

(c) What is the treatment?

Answers

(a) Bilateral Dupuytren's contractures. The left hand is more severe with contracture and flexion of the little finger. The right hand shows early features of thickening and tethering of palmar fascia.

(b) Chronic liver disease, trauma, inherited, idiopathic and epilepsy.

(c) Selective fasciectomy.

Short Case (see Appendix, Figure 13).

It is often bilateral. Initially there is thickening of the palmar fascia then flexion and tethering of the fifth and then fourth fingers occurs. It may be associated with other signs of chronic liver disease (see case 37).

*Baron G. Dupuytren (1777–1835). French surgeon.

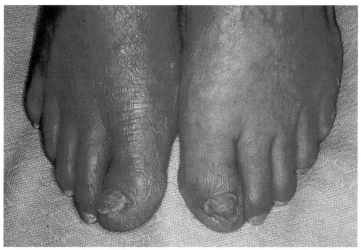

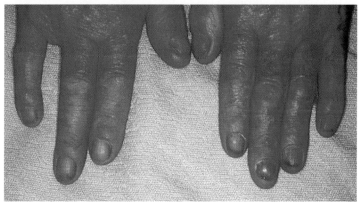

Questions

This man complained of haemoptysis.

(a) Name two abnormalities in these photographs.

(b) What is the diagnosis?

(c) What is the cause of his haemoptysis?

(d) List two other symptoms he may have.

Answers

(a) The nails are thickened and yellow. The right ring finger is absent.
(b) Yellow nail syndrome.
(c) Bronchiectasis.
(d) Swelling of the legs (lymphoedema), breathlessness (bronchiectasis, pleural effusion), wheeze and purulent copious sputum (bronchiectasis).

Discussion

Yellow nail syndrome consists of lymphoedema, pleural effusions (usually chylous), bronchiectasis, sinusitis and yellow nails. The nails become thickened, yellow and dystrophic over time and may be shed. They regrow. It is more common in females and cases are sporadic. The underlying defect is thought to be lymphatic hypoplasia. The reason for the bronchiectasis and sinusitis is not known.

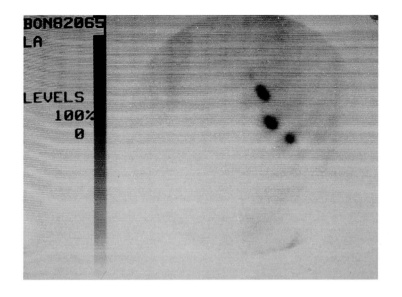

BON82065
LA

LEVELS
100%
0

Questions

This patient had had a stroke.

(a) What is this investigation?

(b) What does it show?

(c) What is the probable cause?

Answers

(a) An isotope bone scan (see case 31).

(b) Three areas of increased uptake due to fractured ribs.

(c) The patient probably fell after the stroke occurred causing the rib fractures.

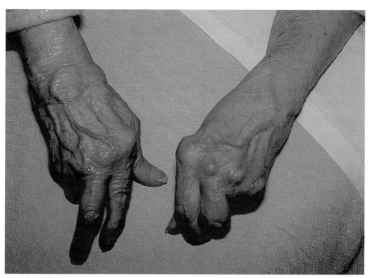

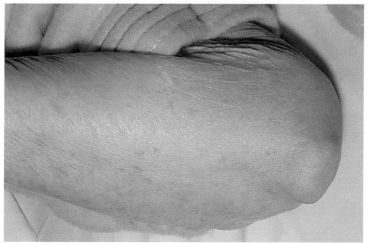

Questions

(a) Name three abnormalities in these photographs.

(b) What is the diagnosis?

(c) What is the treatment?

CASE 56

Answers

(a) Flexion deformities of the fingers, swelling of the metacarpo-phalangeal (MCP) joints with ulnar deviation, Z-shaped deformity of the right thumb, wasting of the small hand muscles, thinning of the skin, swelling of both wrist joints and rheumatoid nodules on the right elbow.

(b) Rheumatoid arthritis (all cases with rheumatoid nodules are seropositive).

(c) Non-steroidal anti-inflammatory drugs (NSAIDs) are the mainstay of treatment. Second-line drugs include gold (side-effects: bone suppression, proteinuria is common, nephrotic syndrome is rare) and penicillamine (side-effects: proteinuria, bone marrow suppression). Systemic steroids and immunosuppressive therapy is rarely needed. Other therapies include surgical techniques, local joint injections with steroids and rehabilitation techniques.

Short Case (see Appendix, Figure 14)

There is a symmetrical deforming arthropathy of the hands involving the MCP joints and proximal interphalangeal (PIP) joints. The distal inter-phalangeal (DIP) joints are spared. There is ulnar deviation of the fingers caused by subluxation of the MCP joints. There may be arteritic lesions in the nail folds. Other signs in the hands include: Z-shaped deformity of the thumb, Boutonnière deformity (flexion deformity of PIP joint and extension of DIP and MCP joints), 'swan neck' deformity (hyperextension of PIP and flexion of MCP and DIP joints) and palmar erythema. Other clinical features to note are:

- Leg ulcers (vasculitic).
- Anaemia (pallor). This is usually normochromic/normocytic but may be iron deficient because of NSAIDs. It may be due to bone marrow failure from drugs (penicillamine, gold) or it may be macrocytic owing to associated pernicious anaemia.
- Cardiovascular system. Pericarditis, mitral regurgitation and aortic regurgitation may be present but all are uncommon.
- Respiratory system. Pleural effusions and pulmonary fibrosis may occur. *Caplan's syndrome involves large rheumatoid nodules in the lungs of coal miners which may coalesce and cavitate.
- Eyes. Episcleritis and scleromalacia perforans may occur. Cataracts occur secondary to steroid therapy.
- Neurological system. Peripheral neuropathy, mononeuritis multiplex and carpal tunnel syndrome are associated.
- Sjogren's syndrome.
- Secondary amyloidosis (macroglossia, hepatosplenomegaly, nephrotic syndrome).

Discussion

Rheumatoid arthritis is more common in women (3:1). It is associated with HLA-DR4. Rheumatoid factor is a circulating IgM antibody to the patient's own IgG. High titres correlate with a severe arthritis and a higher incidence of extra-articular disease. It is also related to a worse prognosis. It is present in 50% of patient with rheumatoid arthritis but 100% of those with rheumatoid nodules and Sjogren's syndrome.

*Felty's syndrome occurs in long-standing rheumatoid arthritis. It consists of rheumatoid arthropathy, splenomegaly, neutropenia (pancytopenia and haemolytic anaemia may be present), lymphadenopathy, skin pigmentation, leg ulceration, keratoconjunctivitis sicca and a positive rheumatoid factor.

Other autoimmune diseases associated with rheumatoid arthritis include hypothryoidism, Graves' disease, pernicious anaemia, diabetes mellitus, Addison's disease, ulcerative colitis, SLE, hypoparathyroidism and primary ovarian failure.

*A. Caplan. British physician.

*A.R. Felty (1895–1964). American physician, Johns Hopkins Medical School, Baltimore, USA.

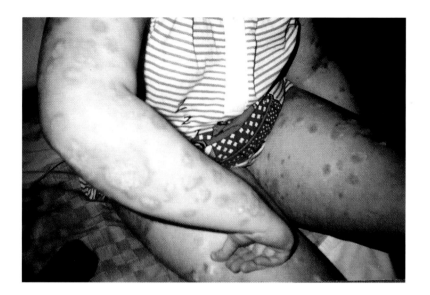

Questions

(a) What is the diagnosis?

(b) Name two other physical signs she may have.

(c) What is the treatment of this condition?

CASE 57

Answers

(a)   Psoriasis.
(b)   Psoriatic arthropathy (asymmetrical arthropathy involving the terminal interphalangeal joints, may mimic rheumatoid arthritis, rheumatoid factor is negative), pitting of the nails and onycholysis.
(c)   Treatment consists of coal tar, dithranol (applied in this patient), local steroids and PUVA (psoralen and UV light). Systemic steroids and anti-metabolites (methotrexate) and orally active vitamin A derivatives (retinoids) are rarely needed.

Short Case

The plaques of psoriasis are most commonly found on the extensor surfaces, behind the ears, in the scalp and navel. Psoriatic arthropathy and nail changes may be present with or without skin lesions. Psoriatic arthropathy may mimic rheumatoid arthropathy (as may the arthropathy associated with scleroderma and SLE, although the latter is rarely erosive or deforming).

Discussion

Psoriasis affects 2% of the population and is familial in 30% of cases. Psoriatic arthropathy occurs in 10% of cases and is associated with nail changes (nail pitting, dystrophic changes, onycholysis). It is seronegative. It may be rapidly progressive and deforming (arthritis mutilans). Sacroiliitis also occurs in 30% of cases.

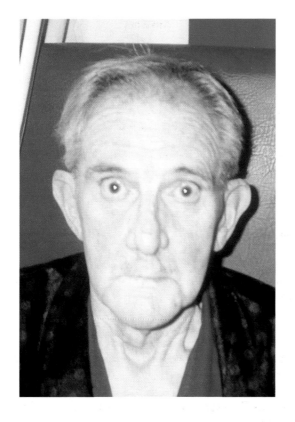

Questions

This man complained of sudden hair loss.

(a) What is the physical sign demonstrated in this photograph?

(b) What is the diagnosis?

Answers

(a) Exophthalmos (and lid retraction).
(b) Thyrotoxicosis (see case 44).

Short Case

Exophthalmos is usually bilateral in association with Graves' disease and is of varying degrees of severity. Exophthalmos means protrusion of the eye with the sclera visible below and above the iris on forward gaze. Other eye signs include lid retraction and lid lag (delay in the upper lid following the eyeball when moving vertically superiorly to inferiorly). There may be periorbital swelling, chemosis, corneal ulceration and ophthalmoplegia in severe cases.

Discussion

Malignant exophthalmos (congestive ophthalmopathy) can cause pain and a risk of blindness because of pressure on the optic nerve. Treatment may include systemic steroids, lateral tarsorrhaphy and orbital decompression. Ophthalmoplegia is due to infiltration, oedema and fibrosis of the external occular muscles. The eye signs are not related to treatment of thyrotoxicosis and progression is unpredictable. Other causes of exophthalmos include:

- **Unilateral** – retro-orbital tumour, cellulitis.
- **Bilateral** – cavernous sinus thrombosis, caroticocavernous fistula.

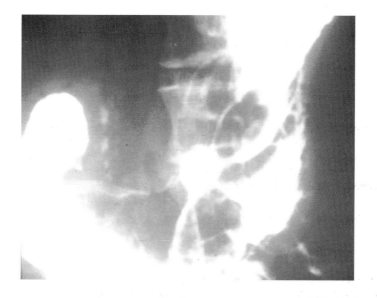

Questions

(a) What is this investigation?

(b) What is the diagnosis?

(c) Name three symptoms the patient may have.

(d) What is the treatment?

Answers

(a) Barium meal.

(b) There is a gastric ulcer on the lesser curve of the stomach.

(c) Epigastric pain (usually precipitated by food), anorexia, nausea, vomiting and weight loss.

(d) All patients should have an endoscopy and biopsy. Treatment is with an H_2 antagonist (e.g. ranitidine 150 mg b.d.) for 6 weeks. A repeat endoscopy should be performed to ensure healing. Ulcers resistant to healing with H_2 antagonists should be treated with a proton pump inhibitor (e.g. Omeprazole 20 mg daily) but careful follow-up is essential so as not to miss a gastric carcinoma.

Discussion

Gastric ulcers on the greater curve of the stomach are more likely to be malignant although lesser curve ulcers can be malignant. About 1% of gastric ulcers become malignant. The patient may complain of more weight loss and dysphagia. Pyloric obstruction may occur. The prognosis is poor and the 5-year survival after surgery is only 20%.

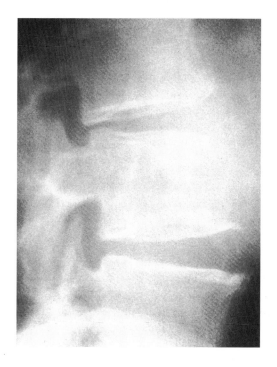

Questions

This 66-year-old man complained of back pain. He had had an episode of haematuria 4 months previously.

(a) What does this X-ray show?

(b) What is the cause in this case?

(c) Name one biochemical abnormality that may be present.

Answers

(a)   Destruction of the vertebral body owing to osteolytic metastases.
(b)   Renal carcinoma (previous haematuria).
(c)   Hypercalcaemia (may produce confusion, polyuria, polydipsia and constipation). The serum alkaline phosphatase level may also be elevated. Haematological abnormalities include anaemia as a result of bone marrow infiltration. This may be normochromic/normocytic or there may be a pancytopenia.

Discussion

Metastases in bone may produce purely osteolytic lesions or an osteoblastic reaction or both. Tumour deposits tend to be predominantly one type. Carcinoma of the kidney nearly always produces osteolytic metastases whereas carcinomas of the prostate and pancreas produce osteoblastic metastases. Other tumours that commonly metastasize to bone are breast, lung and thyroid.

Bone metastases are associated with pain, weakness and anaemia and usually occur in the terminal stages of the disease. Bones may undergo pathological fracture and occasionally patients present with spontaneous fracture. These require internal fixation to control pain. Radiotherapy is also effective in pain control. Non-steroidal anti-inflammatory drugs are particularly useful and slow-release morphine is also used as necessary.

Radionucleotide bone scans are more sensitive in detecting bone metastases than plain X-rays. These are often used for:

- Diagnosing occult metastases.
- Staging disease; for example, in lung carcinoma bone metastases would mean the tumour is inoperable.
- Monitoring treatment.

It should be noted that isotope bone scans can produce false-positives in the following cases: fracture, Paget's disease of the bone, abscesses and osteomalacia.

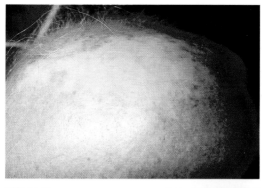

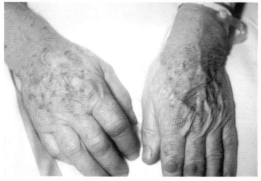

Questions

(a) Describe the abnormalities.

(b) What is the diagnosis?

(c) Name three associated conditions.

Answers

(a) Areas of depigmentation on the dorsum of the hands and scalp.
(b) Vitiligo.
(c) Autoimmune diseases: diabetes mellitus, pernicious anaemia, rheumatoid arthritis (see case 56), Sjögren's syndrome, Graves' disease, hypothyroidism, Addison's disease, systemic sclerosis, dermatomyositis and coeliac disease.

Short Case (see Appendix, Figure 15)

Areas of depigmentation may occur anywhere and may be asymmetrical. If on the hands, look for signs of other related disease (rheumatoid arthritis, systemic sclerosis). If on the face, look for other signs, e.g. heliotrope rash (purplish rash) around the eyes (also on the back of the hands) associated with dermatomyositis. If vitiligo is associated with thyroid disease there may be a 'peaches and cream' complexion, periorbital puffiness or exophthalmos, etc. Systemic sclerosis will be evident if the skin is smooth and shiny, the mouth aperture will be reduced and the nose 'beak-like' and there may be telangiectasia.

Discussion

Vitiligo may occur in sites subject to friction, which are often affected by the Koebner's phenomenon. Alopecia areata and premature greying of the hair are also associated with vitiligo as well as the autoimmune diseases listed above.

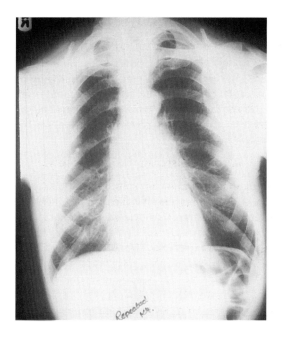

Questions

This is the chest X-ray of a patient who complained of orthopnoea, haemoptysis and dysphagia.

(a) Name two abnormalities on this X-ray.

(b) What is the probable diagnosis?

(c) What is the cause of the patient's three symptoms?

Answers

(a)   The left heart border is straight owing to a prominent left atrial appendage and pulmonary artery (pulmonary hypertension). There are *Kerley B lines present (horizontal lines in lower zones of lungs caused by fluid in the interlobular septa) indicating early left ventricular failure. The heart size is normal or small as a result of the stenosed mitral valve reducing the volume of blood delivered to the left ventricle.

(b)   Mitral stenosis with associated pulmonary hypertension and left ventricular failure.

(c)   The patient has orthopnoea resulting from left ventricular failure. Haemoptysis could be due to a bronchial vein rupture caused by pulmonary hypertension, associated pulmonary emboli, left ventricular failure or bronchitis. The dysphagia is due to a large left atrium pressing on the oesophagus.

Short Case

The patient may have malar flush (sign of pulmonary hypertension). The pulse is of small volume and may be irregularly irregular (atrial fibrillation). The apex beat is not displaced but 'tapping' in character owing to a palpable first heart sound. There will be a left parasternal heave as a result of pulmonary hypertension causing a large right ventricle. The first heart sound is loud and after the second sound there is an opening snap (loud first heart sound and opening snap denote the presence of a pliable valve). This is followed by a mid-diastolic rumbling murmur. There may be pre-systolic accentuation produced by atrial systole if the patient is in sinus rhythm. The more severe the stenosis the closer the opening snap is to the second sound and the longer is the murmur. Listen for associated murmurs: mitral regurgitation and aortic valve murmurs.

Discussion

Mitral stenosis is becoming less common now as rheumatic fever is rarely seen. It does occur in 60% of those who have had rheumatic fever and it is four times as common as rheumatic mitral regurgitation and twice as common as mixed mitral valve disease. It is more common in women (4:1). About one-third of patients give no previous history of rheumatic fever.

The main symptom is dyspnoea. This symptom determines the need for valvotomy or mitral valve replacement. Complications of mitral stenosis are thromboembolism (all patients require lifelong anticoagulation to reduce the risk), atrial fibrillation (40%), left and right heart failure and an increase in the incidence of bacterial endocarditis.

The earliest radiological sign of left ventricular failure is prominent upper lobe veins caused by diversion of blood from oedematous lower zones. The Kerley B line may be seen representing oedema in the alveolar septa. Diffuse shadowing then occurs in a 'butterfly wing' distribution and there may be pleural effusions and an enlarged heart.

*P.J. Kerley (1900–1978). British neurologist.

CASE 63

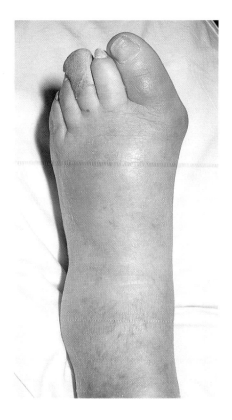

Questions

This patient was receiving treatment for Hodgkin's disease.

(a) What does this photograph show?

(b) What is the diagnosis?

(c) What is the treatment?

163

Answers

(a) There is swelling and erythema of the metatarsophalangeal joint and surrounding erythema over the dorsum of the foot.

(b) Acute gout.

(c) Non-steroidal anti-inflammatory drugs should be used along with allopurinol. Non-steroidal anti-inflammatory drugs need to be continued for at least 6 weeks as allopurinol alone provokes gout by increasing the concentration of monosodium urate crystals in the synovial fluid. Most patients receiving chemotherapy should be commenced on allopurinol routinely to prevent attacks of acute gout. If there are contraindications to non-steroidal anti-inflammatory drugs then colchicine should be used for the acute attack. (See case 7.)

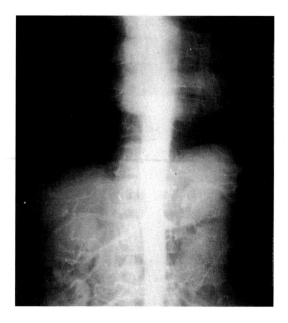

Questions

This 50-year-old man complained of exertional dyspnoea and orthopnoea.

(a) What is this investigation?

(b) What does it show?

(c) What is the cause of his symptoms?

(d) What features would his ECG show?

(e) What is the treatment?

CASE 64

Answers

(a)   A renal arteriogram.
(b)   Left renal artery stenosis.
(c)   Left ventricular failure resulting from prolonged hypertension. Renal artery stenosis is a rare cause of hypertension (<1% of cases).
(d)   Left ventricular hypertrophy/strain pattern.
(e)   Control of blood pressure is essential (angiotensin converting enzyme inhibitors are contraindicated). Dilatation of the renal artery under radiological control (angioplasty) is useful in helping to control blood pressure and in some cases all drugs can be withdrawn. It may also be necessary to improve renal function.

Short Case

The patient will have signs of long-standing hypertension: hypertensive retinopathy; displaced apex beat with thrusting character of left ventricular hypertrophy; there may be signs of left ventricular failure. The diagnosis is suggested by a renal artery bruit. The patient often has signs of vascular disease elsewhere: carotid artery bruits, femoral bruits, impalpable foot pulses, loss of hair on pale legs, etc.

Discussion

The most common cause of renal artery stenosis is atheroma or a combination of atheroma and thrombosis (two-thirds of cases). This usually occurs at the origin of the main renal artery, in its proximal third or at the distal bifurcation of the artery. It usually affects men who are cigarette smokers and who have evidence of vascular disease elsewhere. The remaining cases are due to fibromuscular hyperplasia, which predominantly affects women. The patients are usually younger. There is less involvement of other sites but an association with cigarette smoking has been described. The middle and distal third of the artery is involved and the right side more than the left. The classical arteriogram appearance is like a string of beads but a single stenosed area may be seen.

The reduced renal perfusion in renal artery stenosis results in increased renin secretion by the juxtaglomerular cells resulting in increased angiotensin II, which is a potent vasoconstrictor. Angiotensin II also stimulates the release of aldosterone, which causes sodium retention.

Several investigations may be used in establishing the diagnosis but renal angiography is the most accurate though not without risk. An intravenous urogram classically shows a delayed nephrogram, a small kidney and later hyperconcentration of the dye. Isotope renograms have high false-positive and false-negative rates for diagnosis but are useful to quantify the stenosis and assess renal function (by indirect measurement of glomerular filtration rate).

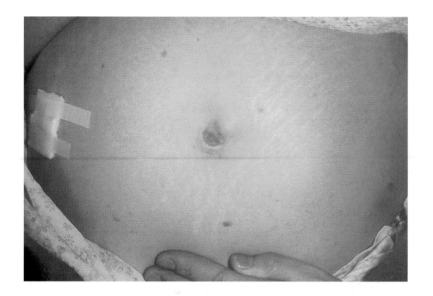

Questions

This 70-year-old woman complained of early satiety and anorexia.

    (a) Name three abnormal features in this photograph.

    (b) What is the cause of these signs?

    (c) What is the most probable underlying diagnosis?

CASE 65

Answers

(a) Abdominal distension and chronic striae, dressing in the right flank, and a nodule at the umbilicus (*Sister Mary Joseph nodule).

(b) There is chronic ascites, which has been tapped (dressing over the peritoneal tap site) for diagnostic purposes. The umbilical nodule is spread of an intra-abdominal tumour, the most common being stomach and ovary.

(c) In view of her symptoms the most likely underlying diagnosis is metastatic carcinoma of the stomach.

Short Case

The patient may be cachectic and have signs of metastatic liver disease: jaundice anaemia and Virchow's node. The abdomen is distended and there may be an epigastric mass. Shifting dullness and a fluid thrill will be evident.

*Sister Mary Joseph Dempsey (1856–1939). Nursing nun, St Mary's Hospital, New York, USA.

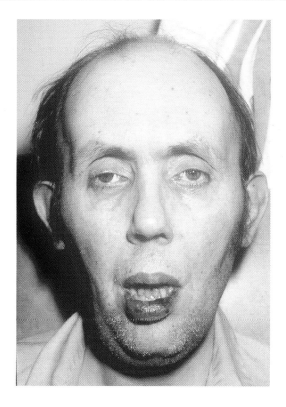

Questions

(a) Name three abnormal features in this photograph.

(b) What is the diagnosis?

(c) What is the inheritance pattern?

(d) What is the treatment?

Answers

(a) Drooping mouth (transverse smile), bilateral ptosis, frontal balding and low set ears.
(b) Dystrophia myotonica.
(c) Autosomal dominant.
(d) Myotonia can be relieved by phenytoin, quinine or procainamide but there is no treatment for the weakness.

Short Case (see Appendix, Figure 16)

The patient has a typical myotonic facies (droopy mouth). There is frontal balding, ptosis and wasting of facial, sternomastoid and shoulder girdle muscles. The quadriceps are involved. The limb reflexes may be decreased or absent. Myotonia (slow relaxation of muscles) is demonstrated by asking to shake the patient's hand. He/she will have difficulty leaving go of your hand. There may be percussion myotonia when indentations made in the tongue or hand muscles take time to disappear owing to slow relaxation. The patient may have dysarrthria as a result of myotonia of the tongue and pharynx. The condition is associated with a decreased intellect.

Fundoscopy may reveal cataract or diabetic retinopathy (diabetes mellitus is associated with this condition). There may be signs associated with a cardiomyopathy (low blood pressure, small volume pulse, signs of cardiac failure).

Discussion

Dystrophia myotonica is more common in males. It becomes more severe in succeeding generations ('anticipation'). The onset of symptoms and signs occurs between 15 and 40 years of age.

There is the classical facial appearance as described. Myotonia is worsened by cold and excitement and reduced by rapid activity. The condition is associated with a cardiomyopathy which may result in heart failure and sudden death from arrhythmias. The patients are of low intellect and are usually impotent and/or sterile (testicular atrophy). There is an association with diabetes mellitus and nodular thyroid gland enlargement. Dysphagia, abdominal pain, hyperventilation and post anaesthetic respiratory failure are common.

Myotonia congenita (*Thomsen's disease) is an autosomal dominant condition which has an earlier onset than dystrophia myotonica. There is myotonia without the other features of dystrophia myotonica and the reflexes are present. The patients present with falls and painless stiffness which is made worse by cold and improved by repeated movements.

*A. J. T. Thomsen (1815–1896). Danish physician.

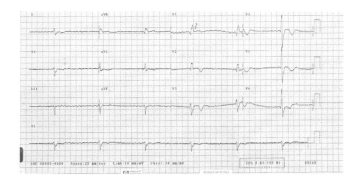

Questions

This 78-year-old man presented with a generalized seizure. He had no previous history of ill health.

(a) Name three abnormalities on the ECG.

(b) What is the possible cause of his convulsion?

(c) List two symptoms the patient may have had.

(d) What is the treatment?

CASE 67

Answers

(a) Atrial fibrillation with a ventricular rate of about 40/minute, left axis deviation (QRS frontal axis is −75°), right bundle branch block, T-wave inversion in leads V1–V6.

(b) His convulsion was probably due to bradycardia/period of asystole causing a decreased cardiac output and cerebral irritation. It may have been due to a cerebral thromboembolism originating from an intracardiac thrombus.

(c) Dizziness, dyspnoea (due to heart failure), syncope (*Stokes–Adams attacks).

(d) A permanent pacemaker.

Discussion

This ECG shows evidence of bifascicular block (right bundle branch block and left axis deviation; right bundle branch block and left anterior fascicular block). The most likely aetiology is ischaemic heart disease (there is T-wave inversion in V1–V6). This type of bifasicular block shown is the most common as the posterior fascicle of the left bundle branch has a better blood supply and is less likely to be affected. Block of the anterior and posterior fascicles of the left bundle branch results in left bundle branch block. Trifascicular block results in AV block. The risk of bifascicular block progressing to trifascicular block is low but is more likely if there is right bundle branch block and left posterior fascicular block.

Syncope resulting from episodes of asystole or ventricular fibrillation has been called a Stokes–Adams attack. The 12-lead ECG could be normal and the diagnosis may be made on a 24-hour ECG. There is no warning before the collapse and during it the patient is pulseless. It may progress to a fit as in this case. On recovery, which is usually quick unless a fit has occurred, there is a vivid flush to the skin. A permanent pacemaker is needed.

*W. Stokes (1804–1878). Irish physician.

*R. Adams (1791–1875). Irish surgeon.

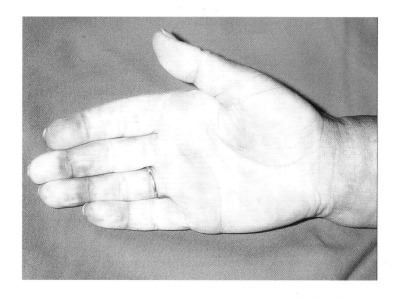

Questions

This woman had difficulty vacuuming the floor as this produced the reaction shown.

(a) What is the diagnosis?

(b) What is the cause in this case?

(c) Name two other causes of this condition.

(d) What is the treatment?

Answers

(a) *Raynaud's phenomenon.
(b) Vibrating instruments, e.g. vacuum cleaner.
(c) Connective tissue disorder (systemic sclerosis, SLE, rheumatoid arthritis, polymyositis), hypothyroidism, idiopathic (usually young females, starts in childhood) and cervical rib.
(d) Remove the precipitating factors, i.e. vibration, cold, cervical rib. Heated gloves may be helpful and nifedipine helps in some cases because of its vasodilatory action.

Short Case

In Raynaud's disease there is an abnormal vascular reactivity. Cold often precipitates the phenomenon. The fingers become white and numb. On recovery they become blue (cyanosis) and then red (rebound hyper-aemia which is painful). In the examination, patients have chronically impaired circulation and may have changes (as in this case) even in a warm environment. It is often shown as a feature of systemic sclerosis in the examination and therefore note other features of this condition.

*M. Raynaud (1834–1881). French physician

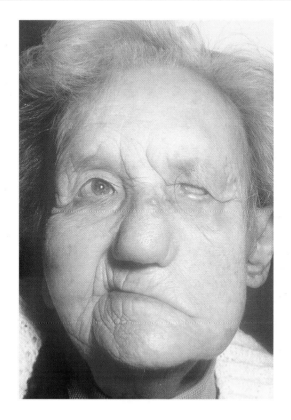

Questions

(a) What is the diagnosis?

(b) Name two possible causes.

Answers

(a)   Left lower motor neurone VIIth cranial palsy.
(b)   *Bell's palsy, Ramsay–Hunt syndrome, cerebropontine meningioma or acoustic neuroma (produces Vth, VIth, VIIth and VIIIth palsies and cerebellar ataxia), middle ear disease, parotid tumour and causes of mononeuritis multiplex.

Short Case

In a lower motor neurone VIIth palsy there is paralysis of the upper and lower face. In an upper motor neurone VIIth palsy (commonest cause of which is a cerebrovascular accident in the carotid artery territory) the function of the upper face is preserved. This is because the frontalis, corrugator superficialis and orbicularis occuli muscles are supplied bilaterally (innervated by both right and left leg VIIth cranial nerves).

Look in the ear for vesicles of herpes zoster (Ramsey–Hunt syndrome, there is also loss of taste to the anterior two thirds of the tongue and vesicles on the palate). There may be scarring if due to middle ear surgery or a parotid tumour (taste is present if the facial nerve is affected after leaving the stylomastoid foramen). Bell's palsy, if severe, may be associated with loss of taste and hyperacusis owing to involvement of the nerve to stapedius (branch of VIIth).

Discussion

Bilateral VIIth nerve palsies may be easily missed as there is no asymmetry. Causes include:

● Guillain–Barré syndrome
● Bilateral Bell's palsy
● Myasthenia gravis
● Sarcoidosis
● Motor neurone disease.

*Sir C. Bell (1774–1842). Scottish physiologist and surgeon.

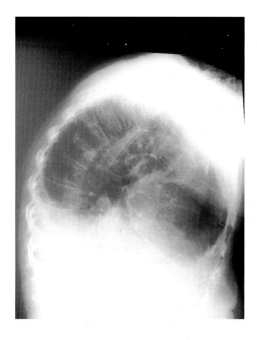

Questions

This 80-year-old woman complained of backache.

(a) Describe the abnormalities in this photograph.

(b) What is the diagnosis?

(c) What is the differential diagnosis?

(d) Name two possible treatments.

Answers

(a) Kyphosis caused by wedge-shaped collapse (crush fracture) of vertebral bodies. There is loss of bone density (osteopenia).

(b) Idiopathic osteoporosis.

(c) It is important to exclude other causes of loss of bone density, i.e. myeloma, secondary carcinoma and thyrotoxicosis particularly in the elderly.

(d) Oestrogens (hormone replacement therapy) prevent bone loss in post-menopausal women and reduce the risk of vertebral and hip fractures. Intermittent cyclical etidronate (given for 2 weeks out of 15) prevents bone loss and reduces the risk of vertebral fractures in older women. Calcitonin prevents bone loss and reduces vertebral and hip fractures but it is expensive. Vitamin D and calcium have been shown to decrease hip fracture rate in the elderly.

Short Case

The patient will have a marked kyphosis ('dowagers hump'). There may be signs of associated disease, e.g. steroid purpura and paper-thin skin. Vertebral collapse can result in spinal cord compression with signs in the lower limbs, e.g. sensory level, paralysis, decreased/absent reflexes.

Discussion

Up to 30% of women and 50% of men with vertebral fractures have secondary osteoporosis (steroids, thyrotoxicosis, Cushing's syndrome, myeloma, hypogonadism in men). Osteoporosis is usually asymptomatic until fractures occur. Fractures of the forearm, (Colles) hip and vertebral bodies occur. Population-based bone density screening is unproven in the prevention of osteoporotic fractures though it may be a useful tool in the management of high-risk individuals.

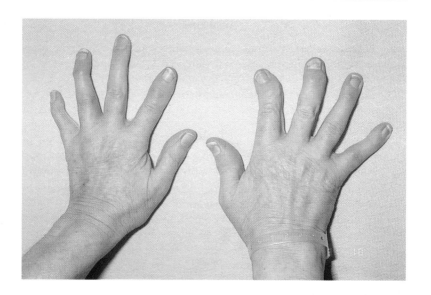

Questions

(a) Name two abnormalities in these hands.

(b) What is the probable diagnosis?

Answers

(a) Onycholysis (right middle finger), *Heberden's nodes (right index and middle finger), subluxed right index DIP joint. There is an early swan neck deformity of the left ring finger.

(b) Psoriatic arthropathy with co-existent osteoarthrosis.

Discussion

Heberden's nodes are osteophytes at the DIP joints. At the PIP joints they are called *Bouchard's nodes. They are a sign of osteoarthrosis and are more common in women. It is thought that a single autosomal gene is involved, which is dominant in females and recessive in males.

Onycholysis is the separation of the nail from its nail bed. The brown discoloration of the nail that results may be due to the accumulation of dirt or infection with *Pseudomonas* which produces a green/black discoloration. Causes of onycholysis include:

- Trauma.
- Psoriasis.
- Infection – fungal, Pseudomonas.
- Yellow nail syndrome (see case 54).
- Hyperthyroidism (Plummer's nails).
- Impaired circulation.
- Drugs – cloxacillin, demeclocycline.

*W. Heberden (1710–1801). English physician.

*C.J. Bouchard (1837–1915). French physician.

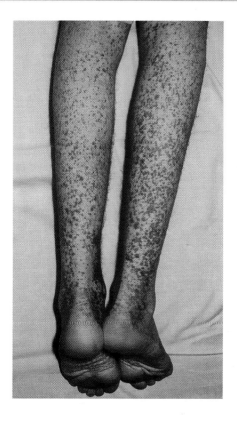

Questions

This 14-year-old boy complained of colicky abdominal pain.

(a) What is shown in this photograph?

(b) What is the diagnosis?

(c) Name two other symptoms he may have.

(d) What is the cause of his abdominal pain?

(e) What is the treatment?

Answers

(a) An extensive purpuric rash on the lower limbs.
(b) *Henoch–Schönlein purpura.
(c) Arthralgia, malaise, rigors, pruritus (due to urticaria) and melaena.
(d) Haemorrhage and oedema of the bowel wall causing intestinal bleeding or intussusception.
(e) Symptomatic and supportive. Corticosteroids are of value in treating the gastrointestinal complications.

Short Case

The short case will be to describe the purpuric rash. There is a polyarthropathy affecting mainly the ankles, knees, hips, wrists and elbows.

Discussion

Henoch-Schönlein (anaphylactoid) purpura occurs in children, more commonly boys. An upper respiratory tract infection precedes 90% of cases but beta haemolytic streptococci are isolated in only 30%. There is a widespread vasculitis involving arteries and capillaries. The purpuric rash classically occurs on the buttocks, ankles and extensor surface. Urticaria of the face and legs occurs. Fever and gastrointestinal bleeding are part of the syndrome. There is a non-migratory polyarthritis of the large joints. Acute proliferative glomerulonephritis presents as proteinuria and haematuria and renal failure is uncommon. The disease is self-limiting lasting about 1 month. The prognosis is good but it may recur. A similar disease in adults carries a worse prognosis.

*E.H. Henoch (1820–1910). German paediatrician.

*J.L. Schönlein (1793–1864). German physician.

CASE 73

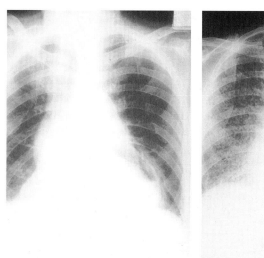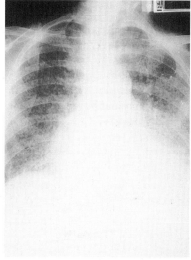

Questions

This 83-year-old woman complained of indigestion. She had had a chest X-ray (left). Six weeks later she was admitted to hospital drowsy and very ill with a blood pressure of 80/40. Her chest X-ray on admission is on the right. She had a history of polymyalgia rheumatica for which she had been taking oral prednisolone for three years.

(a) What was the probable cause of her indigestion?

(b) What abnormalities can be seen on her second chest X-ray?

(c) What is the differential diagnosis of the appearance of the second chest X-ray?

(d) What is the diagnosis in this case ?

Answers

(a)   A hiatus hernia. This can be seen on the first chest X-ray (fluid level behind the heart shadow).

(b)   There is widespread miliary shadowing.

(c)   The causes of widespread diffuse shadowing on a chest X-ray are: miliary tuberculosis, sarcoidosis, lymphangitis carcinomatosa, pneumoconiosis, rheumatoid arthritis, systemic sclerosis, SLE, histiocytosis X, histioplasmosis, radiation pneumonitis and drugs (nitrofurantoin, busulphan, paraquat).

(d)   Miliary tuberculosis. Owing to her age she was also immuno-suppressed on steroids.

Short case (see Appendix, Figure 17)

There may be no physical signs in the lungs and in fact the chest X-ray is normal in 50% of cases. There are bilateral crackles in the late stages. Hepatosplenomegaly occurs and choroidal tubercles should be sought on ophthalmoscopy.

Discussion

Disseminated tuberculosis is difficult to diagnosis in the elderly and it is sometimes called 'cryptic' or 'concealed' tuberculosis. The diagnosis is made late or at post-mortem examination. The elderly are more susceptible to reactivation of old infection because of decreased cell mediated immunity that occurs with ageing. Symptoms are non-specific, most commonly anorexia and weight loss. Pyrexia is common. There is often hyponatraemia (due to inappropriate ADH secretion) and disturbed liver function tests (most commonly an elevated alkaline phosphatase). There may be a pancytopenia because of bone marrow involvement. Tuberculin tests may be negative. Initial treatment consists of quadruple anti-tuberculous therapy and treatment should continue for 6 months. Oral corticosteroids may be useful when given in conjunction with anti-tuberculous drugs in that they reduce the local inflammatory reaction and decrease systemic upset. The use of steroids and anti-tuberculous drugs should be closely monitored.

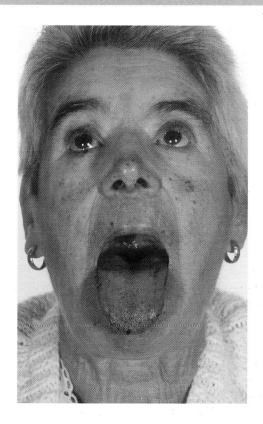

Questions

This woman complained of exertional dyspnoea and palpitations.

(a) What is the physical sign shown?

(b) What is the diagnosis?

(c) What is the inheritance pattern?

(d) What is the cause of her symptoms?

(e) What is the treatment?

(f) Why may she be centrally cyanosed?

Answers

(a)   Telangiectasia on the lips, tongue and face.

(b)   Hereditary haemorrhagic telangectasia (*Osler–Weber–Rendu syndrome).

(c)   Autosomal dominant.

(d)   Chronic iron deficiency anaemia.

(e)   Chronic oral iron therapy. Oestrogens may reduce bleeding by causing squamous metaplasia of the affected mucosa, but side-effects (gynaecomastia and feminization) are unacceptable, particularly in males.

(f)   Due to the presence of an associated large pulmonary arterio-venous aneurysm/fistula. This also results in finger clubbing (may be unilateral).

Short Case (see Appendix, Figure 18)

There are telangiectasia on the mouth, tongue, lips, face, hands and nasal mucosa. The patient may be clinically anaemic (pallor, brittle nails, koilynychia, etc.). In some patients there is associated pulmonary arterio-venous fistulae which result in central cyanosis and finger clubbing.

Discussion

The patient presents with epistaxis (commonest form of presentation), haemoptysis or gastrointestinal bleeding. The patient may have symptoms of chronic iron deficiency anaemia (tiredness, dyspnoea, palpitations). Treatment is with transfusions, if necessary and surgery may be needed if gastrointestinal bleeding is severe. All patients should receive lifelong oral iron therapy. Oestrogens may help to reduce bleeding but side-effects are unacceptable.

*Sir W. Osler (1849–1919). Canadian professor of medicine.

*H.J.L. Rendu (1844–1902). French physician.

*F.P. Weber (1863–1962). British physician.

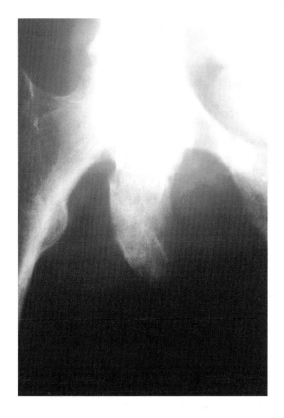

Questions

(a) What abnormality can be seen on this X-ray?

(b) What is the diagnosis?

(c) Name two relevant abnormal blood tests.

(d) List two symptoms the patient may have.

Answers

(a) A *Looser's zone (pseudofracture, *Milkman fracture) in the superior pubic ramus.
(b) Osteomalacia.
(c) Reduced serum phosphate and calcium and increased alkaline phosphatase.
(d) Pain over the pseudofracture. Generalized bone pain is common. Proximal myopathy (waddling gait, unable to get upstairs or comb hair, etc.).

Short Case

In adults the main physical sign of osteomalacia is proximal myopathy. Hypocalcaemic tetany may be demonstrated by provoking carpopedal spasm with the sphygmomanometer set at a level higher than systolic blood pressure (*main d'accoucheur*). This is *Trousseau's sign. Twitching of the facial muscles occurs with hypocalcaemia if the facial nerve is tapped just anterior to the ear. This is *Chvostek's sign. In children other signs are relevant (bow legs, deformity of the chest and skull).

There may be signs of the underlying cause, e.g. malabsorption (abdominal distension, cachexia, pallor, glossitis (iron and vitamin B deficiency), oedema (hypoproteinaemia), bruising (vitamin K deficiency) and signs of subacute combined degeneration of the cord (B_{12} deficiency very rare). Clubbing is associated with some causes of malabsorption, e.g. inflammatory bowel disease, coeliac disease and chronic liver disease.

Discussion

Osteomalacia is due to inadequate mineralization of bone. Causes include:

- Reduced vitamin D intake (dietary and absent sunlight).
- Malabsorption.
- Vitamin D resistance, e.g. chronic renal failure.
- Increased vitamin D metabolism, e.g. chronic anti-convulsant therapy.

Biochemically there is decreased serum levels of phosphate and calcium, raised alkaline phosphatase and a reduced urinary calcium with mild renal tubular acidosis. There is secondary hyperparathyroidism as a result of decreased calcium levels. The Looser's zones seen on X-rays (best seen on the pubic rami, spines scapulae, necks of humerus and femur) are band-like areas of demineralization. They are 'pseudofractures' and result in pain and tenderness.

The management consists of treating the underlying cause, vitamin D and calcium supplementation depending on the aetiology.

*E. Looser (1877–1936). Swiss surgeon.

*L.A. Milkman (1895–1951). American radiologist.

*A. Trousseau (1801–1867). French physician.

*F. Chvosek (1835–1884). Austrian surgeon.

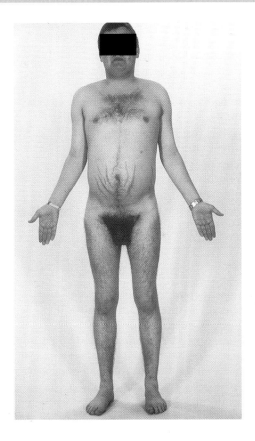

Questions

This patient complained of polydipsia.

(a) What abnormalities can be seen?

(b) What is the cause of his symptom?

(c) What is the diagnosis?

(d) Name two causes of this condition.

CASE 76

Answers

(a) Truncal obesity and abdominal striae.
(b) Diabetes mellitus (occurs in 10% of cases).
(c) *Cushing's syndrome.
(d) (i) Iatrogenic – this is the most common cause, i.e. exogenous prednisolone/ACTH administration.
   (ii) Basophil (or chromophobe) adenoma of the pituitary (Cushing's disease).
   (iii) Adrenocortical adenoma (MEA type I).
   (iv) Adrenocortical carcinoma.
   (v) Ectopic ACTH production, e.g. oat cell carcinoma of bronchus, bronchial adenoma, carcinoid tumour and tumours of thymus, pancreas and ovary.

Short Case

The most common cause of Cushing's syndrome is iatrogenic and there may be signs relevant to the condition under treatment: rheumatoid arthritis, pulmonary fibrosis, chronic asthma.

The patient has a moon face with acne, buffalo hump and truncal obesity. The skin may be bruised with pink/purple striae of the abdomen. Females will be hirsute and males may have gynaecomastia. There may be evidence of pigmentation, which is associated with the ectopic ACTH syndrome. Proximal myopathy may be present.

Discussion

Cushing's syndrome is due to excess production of glucocorticoids producing impaired glucose tolerance and excess mineralocorticoids producing salt retention and hypertension (60% of cases). There is a tendency to hypernatraemia, hypokalaemia (hypokalaemic alkalosis) and glycosuria in most cases (10% have diabetes mellitus). Other features include osteoporosis and vertebral collapse (50%), renal stones (20%) and mental disturbance (depression, mania).

Investigations may include estimation of plasma cortisol levels which show a loss of diurnal variation, serum ACTH level, dexamethasone suppression test (determines whether it is pituitary or adrenal dependent Cushing's syndrome) and a CT scan to establish evidence of pituitary tumour.

Hypophysectomy is the treatment of choice for Cushing's disease. When bilateral adrenalectomy is performed to treat this, *Nelson's syndrome may result (hyperpigmentation caused by excess melanocyte-stimulating hormone (MSH) and ACTH). If there is an adrenal lesion then adrenalectomy is required. Ectopic ACTH syndromes are treated by removing the secreting tumour.

*__H.W. Cushing__ (1869–1939). American neurosurgeon.

*__D.H. Nelson__ (1925–   ). American endocrinologist.

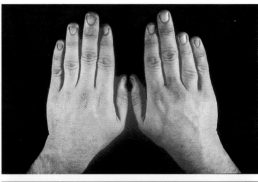

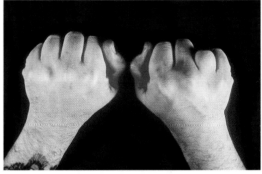

Questions

This patient complained of paraesthesiae in the hands and around the mouth.

(a) What is the physical sign shown?

(b) What is the diagnosis?

(c) Name two other physical signs associated with this condition.

(d) Name two other syndromes in which this physical sign may be present.

(e) What is the cause of the patient's symptoms?

(f) Name one biochemical abnormality.

(g) What abnormality may be seen on skull X-ray?

Answers

(a) A short right fourth metacarpal.
(b) Pseudohypoparathyroidism.
(c) Short stature, obesity and moon face. The patient is also mentally retarded.
(d) Turner's syndrome and Noonan's syndrome.
(e) Hypocalcaemia. Trousseau's sign and Chvostek's sign (see case 75) may be present.
(f) Hypocalcaemia and hyperphosphataemia. The alkaline phosphatase level is normal. Serum parathyroid hormone (PTH) level is high.
(g) Basal ganglia calcification. This is also seen in hypoparathyroidism and it may be familial.

Discussion

Pseudohypoparathyroidism is a rare inherited condition associated with peripheral resistance to PTH. The biochemical changes are the same as hypoparathyroidism but there is a raised PTH level. There is resistance to injected PTH with a failure of the marked rise of urinary phosphate and cyclic AMP seen in true hypoparathyroidism (*Ellsworth–Howard test).

Hypoparathyroidism may be secondary to thyroid surgery or primary (idiopathic) when it is associated with other autoimmune disease (Addison's disease, pernicious anaemia, diabetes mellitus, etc.). Patients may present with signs of hypocalcaemia, e.g. paraesthesiae, muscle twitching, stridor and convulsions. There is an increased incidence of cutaneous moniliasis. There is an association with cataracts and there may be papilloedema. As well as basal ganglia calcification, other soft tissues may have evidence of this.

Treatment in an emergency requires intravenous 10% calcium gluconate. Long-term therapy includes vitamin D and/or calcium supplements.

*R.E. Ellsworth. American physician

*J.E. Howard. American physician.

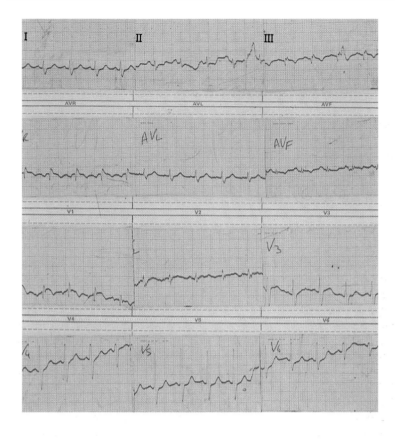

Questions

(a) Describe two abnormalities on this ECG.

(b) What is the diagnosis?

(c) How would you confirm the diagnosis?

CASE 78

Answers

(a) S1 Q3 T3 pattern. Right bundle branch block pattern.
(b) Pulmonary embolus.
(c) An isotope lung scan will show areas of decreased perfusion which are normally ventilated (ventilation/perfusion mismatch). A pulmonary angiogram is more accurate but not without risk. See case 13.

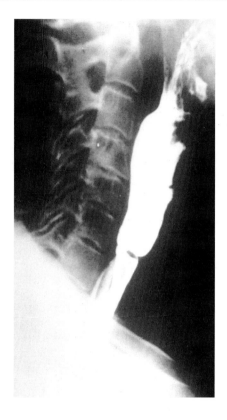

Questions

(a) What is the radiological sign on this barium swallow?

(b) What symptom may the patient have?

(c) What is the diagnosis?

Answers

(a) Post-cricoid oesophageal web.

(b) Dysphagia.

(c) *Plummer–Vinson (*Paterson–Brown-Kelly) syndrome. This iron deficiency anaemia usually occurs in middle-aged females and is associated with dysphagia and a radiologically demonstrable web in the post-cricoid region. They appear as filling defects arising from the anterior wall of the oesophagus just below the cricopharyngeus muscle, seen when the oesophagus is distended with barium. The webs can occur without anaemia and they may precede the development of a post-cricoid carcinoma.

Short Case

The patient may have signs of iron deficiency anaemia: pallor, brittle nails, koilonychia, glossitis, angular stomatitis. There may be causes of iron deficiency anaemia that are clinically apparent, e.g. hereditary haemorrhagic telangiectasia, mass in the right iliac fossa secondary to caecal carcinoma, or suprapubic mass due to fibroids causing menorrhagia.

*H.S. Plummer (1874–1936). American physician.

*P.P. Vinson (1890–1959). American physician.

*D.R. Patterson (1863–1939). British ENT surgeon.

*A. Brown-Kelly (1865–1941). British ENT surgeon.

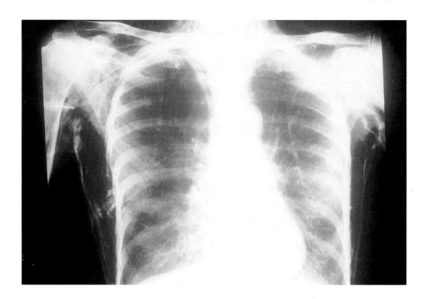

Questions

This 35-year-old man had been repeatedly vomiting after celebrating at a stag party.

(a) What abnormality can be seen on his chest X-ray?

(b) What further radiological procedure is now required?

(c) What is the diagnosis?

(d) What other symptoms will he develop?

(e) Name two other causes of this chest X-ray appearance.

Answers

(a) Extensive surgical (subcutaneous) emphysema.
(b) Gastrografin swallow.
(c) Ruptured oesophagus. This is uncommon but can occur after repeated vomiting. It is more commonly associated with oesophageal tumours.
(d) He may become breathless owing to an associated pneumothorax. Symptoms of oesophageal rupture are those of mediastinitis including severe chest pain and systemic upset. If untreated, septic shock rapidly results in death.
(e) Following a pneumothorax (accidental removal of an intercostal drain), during surgical (cardiothoracic) procedures, stab wounds or asthma (ruptured alveoli may cause a pneumomediastinum which tracks up the neck causing surgical emphysema).

Short Case

There is obvious swelling of the upper torso and face. The eyes may be closed if severe. Palpation will produce a 'crackly' sensation as a result of air in the subcutaneous tissues. There may be signs of an underlying apical pneumothorax: reduced expansion, tracheal displacement to the opposite side, normal or hyper-resonance percussion note, reduced breath sounds, reduced vocal resonance.

Discussion

Treatment for a ruptured oesosphagus includes supportive measures: intravenous fluids and broad-spectrum intravenous antibiotics. Surgical correction is also required. Subcutaneous emphysema is gradually absorbed and resolves spontaneously.

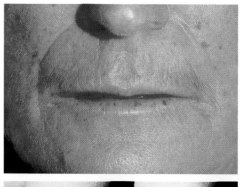

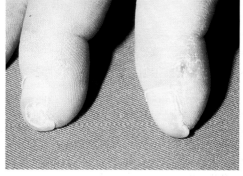

Questions

This woman complained of steatorrhoea.

(a) What physical signs are shown?

(b) What is the cause of her steatorrhoea?

(c) What other gastrointestinal symptoms may she have (name three)?

(d) What is the diagnosis?

Answers

(a) Telangiectasia on the lips and around the mouth and subcutaneous calcinosis (tip of the index finger and nail bed of the middle finger).

(b) Malabsorption. This is due to hypomotility and dilatation of the second part of the duodenum resulting in small bowel bacterial overgrowth. Colonic diverticula are also associated with this condition.

(c) Dysphagia. This is present in up to 90% of cases and is due to oesophageal hypomotility. It may also be due to peptic stricture formation as there is incompetence of the lower oesophageal sphincter resulting in reflux oesophagitis. This also produces symptoms of heartburn.

(d) Systemic sclerosis (scleroderma).

Short Case

The patient is usually a middle-aged female and has a typical facial appearance; smooth, shiny, tight skin giving a 'beaked' nose. The mouth is of small aperture. The skin is pigmented and there is telangiectasia. The hands show similar skin changes (sclerodactyly) and the nails are atrophic. There may be evidence of Raynaud's phenomenon (See case 68) and subcutaneous calcinosis and vitiligo. There may be asymmetrical polyarthropathy which may mimic rheumatoid disease, but this is uncommon.

Examination of the respiratory system may reveal signs of pulmonary fibrosis or overspill pneumonitis. Involvement of the cardiovascular system (cardiomyopathy) may produce signs of heart failure, but this is uncommon.

Discussion

As well as the systems involved above there is often progressive renal failure. Malignant hypertension may result and if not adequately treated this is rapidly fatal. There are sub-types and overlap syndromes described in systemic sclerosis:

- **Crest syndrome** – the pattern consists of Calcinosis, Raynaud's phenomenon, oEsophageal involvement, Sclerodactyly and Telangiectasia. This form progresses slowly and is associated with an overall good prognosis. It is associated with the presence of an anti-centromere antibody which provides a usual diagnostic and prognostic aid.

- **Thibierge–Weissenbach syndrome** – subcutaneous calcification and acrosclerosis.
- **Morphoea** – localized, indurated scleroedematous lesions on the trunk, neck or extremities. This is benign and rarely proceeds to systemic sclerosis.
- **Mixed connective tissue disease** – this is an overlap syndrome combining the features of systemic sclerosis, systemic lupus erythematosis and dermatomyositis. Antibodies to ribonucleoprotein (RNP) are present and DNA antibodies are absent. The prognosis is better than the diseases alone and is steroid responsive.

The management of systemic sclerosis is essentially symptomatic. Steroids are usually ineffective. The 5-year survival is about 70%.

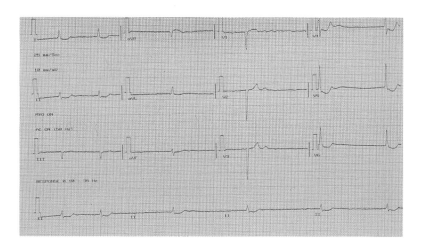

Questions

(a) What is the QRS frontal axis on this ECG?

(b) Name two abnormalities.

(c) What is the diagnosis?

(d) List four symptoms the patient may have.

Answers

(a)   −15°

(b)   Slow atrial fibrillation (ventricular rate <40 per minute) and ST depression ('inverted tick' appearance) V4–V6. There is also poor R-wave progression.

(c)   Digoxin toxicity.

(d)   The patient may feel dizzy owing to the bradycardia. Digoxin toxicity can also produce paroxysms of atrial tachycardia and ventricular tachycardia and this may precipitate angina and heart failure. Other effects of digoxin toxicity are anorexia, nausea, vomiting, diarrhoea, confusion and visual disturbance (xanthopsia – a yellow halo around objects).

Discussion

Digoxin slows conduction at the AV node and is used to control the ventricular rate in atrial fibrillation. It is also an effective oral positively inotropic agent in both atrial fibrillation and sinus rhythm. Digoxin toxicity is common and has been found in 10% of hospital admissions. Toxicity is more likely with renal impairment, hypokalaemia and hypomagnesaemia. Patients who are hypothyroid are sensitive to digoxin. Some drugs, e.g. quinidine, amiodarone and verapamil, increase digoxin levels and produce toxicity.

Treatment of digoxin toxicity consists of withdrawing the drug, correcting electrolyte abnormalities and inserting a temporary pacing wire if required. Tachyarrhythmias may be treated with specific anti-arrhythmic agents. Lignocaine is used for ventricular tachycardia but phenytoin is particularly effective for ventricular tachycardia associated with digoxin toxicity. Cardioversion in the presence of digoxin toxicity can cause dangerous ventricular arrhythmias. It should be the last resort and lignocaine 100 mg intravenously should be given before it is attempted. Cardioversion is safe in the presence of therapeutic levels of digoxin. Digibind (given intravenously) is a digoxin specific antibody. It was specifically designed to treat digoxin overdose, but is expensive.

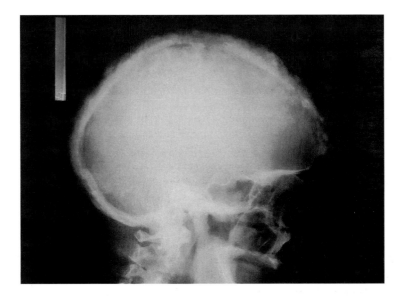

Questions

(a) What is the diagnosis?

(b) What specific symptoms may this patient have (list two)?

(c) Name two abnormal biochemical tests.

(d) Name two possible abnormalities on fundoscopy.

Answers

(a) *Paget's disease of the skull (increased size and thickness of bone with mottled appearance).

(b) Headache (bone pain), deafness (due to compression of the VIIIth cranial nerve and involvement of the ear ossicles) and basilar invagination, which may cause brain stem symptoms and signs.

(c) Raised serum alkaline phosphatase and hypercalcaemia if the patient is immobilized. The 24-hour urinary hydroxyproline is also raised, and this and the serum alkaline phosphatase correlate with the severity of disease and are used in its monitoring.

(d) Optic atrophy and angioid streaks in the retina.

Short Case (see Appendix, Figures 19 and 20)

There may be typical enlargement of the skull and the patient may be wearing a hearing aid. There may be bowing of the tibia and kyphosis (caused by vertebral involvement). Vertebral involvement can lead to spinal stenosis with lower limb signs of spinal cord compression. Basilar invagination can produce brain stem signs.

Discussion

Paget's disease (osteitis deformans) is characterized by increased bone resorption associated with abnormal new bone formation. It mainly affects the axial skeleton and limbs. It is rare in the hands and feet. It is more common in men, affecting 1% of the population after 50 years of age and it has a familial incidence.

Radiologically the normal trabeculae are replaced by coarse irregular striae. This gives a hazy, opaque, mottled appearance. The skull bones may be three to four times the normal thickness. Sometimes large areas of resorption occur in the skull bone (osteoporosis circumscripta).

The main symptom is bone pain. Complications of Paget's disease include:

- Bone deformity and pathological fractures.
- Deafness and basilar invagination.
- High output cardiac failure.
- Urolithiasis (secondary to hypercalcaemia with immobilization).
- Sarcomatous change (<1% of cases).
- Osteoarthrosis of related joints.

Apart from analgesics, specific drugs used in treatment include calcitonin, disodium etidronate and mithramycin.

*Sir James Paget (1814–1899). British surgeon.

CASE 84

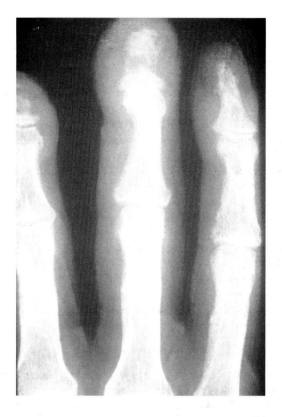

Questions

This patient complained of severe colicky abdominal pain. She had microscopic haematuria.

(a) Name two abnormalities in this X-ray.

(b) What is the diagnosis?

(c) What is the probable cause of her abdominal pain?

(d) List two other symptoms she may have.

CASE 84

Answers

(a) Subperiosteal erosions of the phalanges (commonest on the radial aspect of the middle phalanx) and erosion of the digital terminal tufts (may give the appearance of finger clubbing).
(b) Hyperparathyroidism.
(c) Renal colic.
(d) Hypercalcaemia may cause anorexia, nausea, vomiting, polyuria, polydipsia, constipation and muscle fatigue. Psychiatric symptoms (depression and confusion) occur in 3% of cases.

Short Case

Clinically hypercalcaemia may cause hypotonicity and calcium deposition in the conjunctiva. The hand X-ray appearances occur in 30% of cases. There is osteoporosis as a result of widespread pathological resorption of bone. The skull may show marked osteoporosis ('pepperpot' appearance). An X-ray of the teeth may show loss of the lamina dura of their surrounding bone. Bone cysts resulting from osteoplastic proliferation may develop late in the disease (osteitis fibrosa cystica) and bone deformities can occur.

Discussion

Parathyroid hormone (PTH) increases serum calcium by increasing calcium absorption, increasing calcium mobilization from bone and decreasing renal calcium excretion. There are three types of hyperparathyroidism:
- **Primary** – due to adenoma (85%) hyperplasia of the parathyroid glands (MEA I and II) or parathormone-related hormone production by a tumour, e.g. squamous cell carcinoma of the bronchus.
- **Secondary** – physiological response to hypocalcaemia produced by another disease, e.g. chronic renal failure.
- **Tertiary** – chronic secondary hyperparathyroidism may result in an autonoymous adenoma.

The clinical presentation is as described above. Dyspepsia and peptic ulceration are also more common as PTH increases gastrin levels. Treatment is necessary if there are significant symptoms or bone changes. Surgical resection of the adenoma is required.

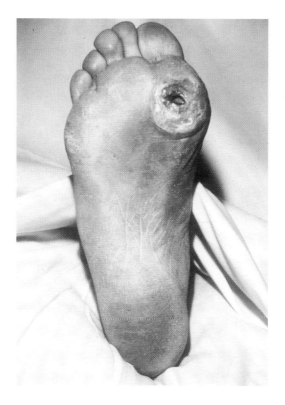

Questions

A chiropodist alerted this patient to this lesion.

    (a) What is the diagnosis?

    (b) Name three possible causes.

Answers

(a) A neuropathic ulcer. It is very deep (head of metatarsals are visible) and yet is painless, as he was not aware of it until the chiropodist mentioned it.

(b) Diabetes mellitus, tabes dorsalis, amyloidosis and leprosy.

Short Case (see Appendix, Figure 21)

The patient will have a peripheral neuropathy (impaired touch, vibration, pain and joint position) in a 'stocking and glove' distribution. Other causes of peripheral neuropathy may result in a neuropathic ulcer. (See case 17)

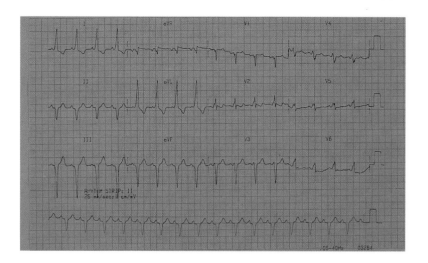

Questions

(a) What is the diagnosis?

(b) Name two complications.

Answers

(a) *Wolff–Parkinson–White syndrome type B.
(b) Paroxysmal supraventricular tachycardia and atrial fibrillation (less common).

Discussion

This is characterized by a short PR interval, a broad QRS complex due to the presence of a delta wave, and a tendency to paroxysmal tachycardia. It affects 1.5 per 1000 of the population. It is caused by an accessory piece of tissue (which is ordinary myocardium) (bundle of Kent) between the atrial and ventricular myocardium which is congenital.

The syndrome is classified into two types depending on the ventricular complex in lead V1. If predominantly positive it is type A and if negative, type B. In type A the bundle of Kent is usually on the left of the heart and in type B it is usually on the right.

The supraventricular tachycardias are treated with the usual anti-arrhythmics except both digoxin and verapamil can actually increase the frequency of conduction in the bundle of Kent and lead to a faster ventricular rate and therefore should be avoided. Surgical division of the bundle of Kent may be required if drugs are ineffective or cannot be tolerated. In the young, radiofrequency ablation of the accessory bundle should be considered.

*L. Wolff (1898–1972). American physician.

*J. Parkinson (1885–1976). English physician.

*P.D. White (1886–1973). American physician.

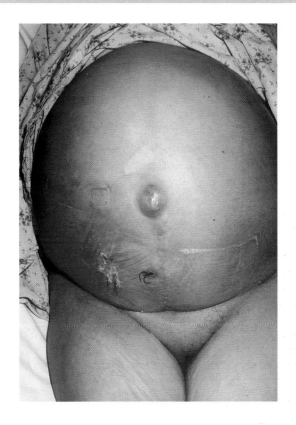

Questions

(a) Name three abnormalities in this photograph.

(b) What is the cause?

Answers

(a)   Abdominal distension (ascites), caput medusae and a stitch from a previous peritoneal tap.

(b)   Portal hypertension.

Short Case

There may be other signs of chronic liver disease (See cases 37 and 53).

Discussion

Causes of portal hypertension are:

- **Pre-hepatic** (20% of cases). Thrombosis of portal vein (congenital), congenital absence of portal vein, portal lymphadenopathy (lymphoma, carcinoma).
- **Intrahepatic** (80% of cases). Cirrhosis, schistosomiasis, sarcoidosis, Hodgkin's disease, veno-occlusive (Bush tea disease).
- **Post-hepatic** (rare). Constrictive pericarditis, Budd-Chiari syndrome.

The lower oesophagus, umbilicus, lower third of rectum and anal canal and subdiaphragmatic and retroperitoneal areas are sites of portacaval anastamoses. Varices in these areas develop when portal hypertension is severe.

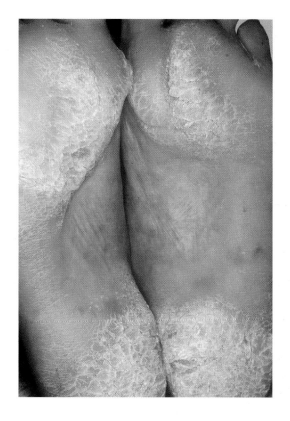

Questions

This 50-year-old man complained of dysphagia.

(a) What is the abnormality?

(b) What is the cause of his dysphagia?

(c) What is the diagnosis?

(d) What is the inheritance pattern of this condition?

Answers

(a) Plantar hyperkeratosis.
(b) Oesophageal carcinoma.
(c) Tylosis.
(d) Autosomal dominant.

Discussion

Tylosis is a rare condition in which plantar and palmar hyperkeratosis is associated with oesophageal carcinoma (45% of cases). Patients and families should be screened by having regular endoscopies to detect early carcinoma.

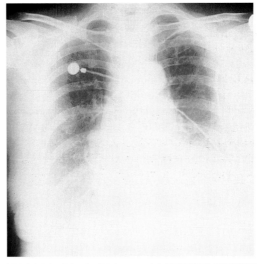

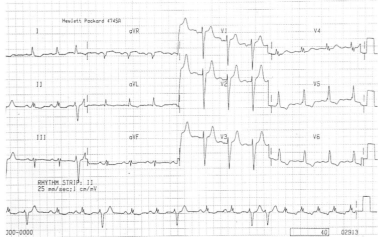

Questions

This chest X-ray and ECG belong to the same patient.

(a) What does the chest X-ray show?

(b) What does the ECG show?

(c) List three causes of the ECG appearance.

Answers

(a)   Cardiomegaly, left pleural effusion and interstitial oedema (radiological signs of left ventricular failure).

(b)   Left bundle branch block. There are a few ventricular premature (ectopic) beats but the presence of left bundle branch block makes further interpretation of the ECG difficult.

(c)   Causes of left bundle branch block are: ischaemic heart disease, systemic hypertension, aortic valve disease, cardiomyopathy and myocarditis.

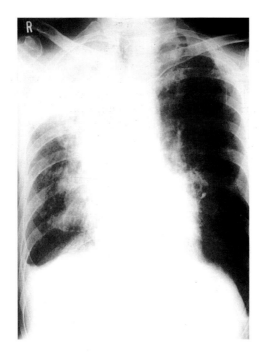

Questions

This 50-year-old Irish man presented with a cough. He was an insulin-dependent diabetic.

(a) What abnormalities can be seen on the chest X-ray?

(b) What is the likely diagnosis?

(c) What is the treatment?

Answers

(a) Right apical consolidation with deviation of the trachea to the right and a small right pleural effusion.
(b) Tuberculosis (more common in Ireland and in diabetics).
(c) Quadruple therapy (isoniazid, rifampicin, ethambutol and pyrazinamide) for two months, then isoniazid and rifampicin is continued for 4 months. Multiple therapy is required as resistance is common. Sputum sensitivity should be obtained.

Short Case

The patient will have signs of 'old' tuberculosis in the examination situation. There may be signs of apical fibrosis (decreased expansion, tracheal deviation, dullness to percussion, late inspiratory crackles) or bronchiectasis (crackles, finger clubbing), which are complications of previous tuberculous infection. There may be evidence of a previous thoracoplasty before anti-tuberculous drugs were available.

Discussion

The organism is usually *Mycobacterium tuberculosis*. Early symptoms are nonspecific: anorexia, weight loss, fatigue. This is followed by cough, haemoptysis, pleuritic pain and dyspnoea. Erythema nodosum may occur.

Radiologically, activity is suggested by changing 'soft' shadows, progressive apical lesions and cavitation. The tuberculin test may be negative (especially in the elderly) and sputum culture may be negative. If clinical suspicion is strong enough patients should be commenced on anti-tuberculous drugs.

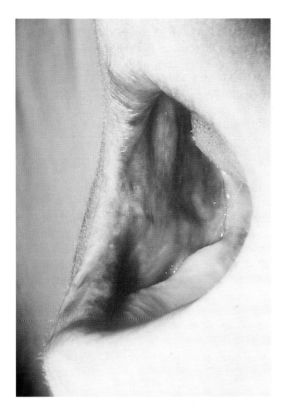

Questions

(a) What is the abnormality in this photograph?

(b) Describe two abnormal blood tests the patient may have.

(c) What is the diagnosis?

(d) What is the treatment?

Answers

(a) Pigmentation of buccal mucosa and lips.
(b) Low serum sodium, high potassium, high urea and low blood sugar. Plasma ACTH is high.
(c) *Addison's disease.
(d) Maintenance therapy with hydrocortisone 20 mg mane, 10 mg nocte and fludrocortisone 0.1 mg mane.

Short Case (see Appendix, Figure 22)

There is generalized pigmentation (due to ACTH stimulating melanocytes, more marked at pressure points, skin creases, buccal mucosa and scars). Vitiligo occurs in 15% of cases. There may be signs of other associated autoimmune disease such as hypothyroidism, Graves' disease or diabetes mellitus. If the hypoadrenalism is secondary there may be signs of the primary disease, e.g. amyloidosis (macroglossia, hepatosplenomegaly, peripheral neuropathy) or haemochromatosis (hepatosplenomegaly). If untreated there will be postural hypotension (systolic drop of $\geq$ 20 mmHg and/or diastolic drop of $\geq$ 10 mmHg). The differential diagnosis is Nelson's syndrome (adrenalectomy scar, bi-temporal hemianopia).

Discussion

Causes of hypoadrenalism are:
- Autoimmune – Addison's disease (HLA-B8 and HLA-DW3). Associated with other autoimmune diseases.
- Hypopituitarism.
- Infiltrations – secondary carcinoma, lymphoma, haemachromatosis, amyloidosis, tuberculosis, histoplasmosis.

Serum electrolytes are abnormal in an impending crisis. The short Synacthen test is positive (no increase in plasma cortisol after tetracosactrin).

*T. Addison (1793–1860). British physician.

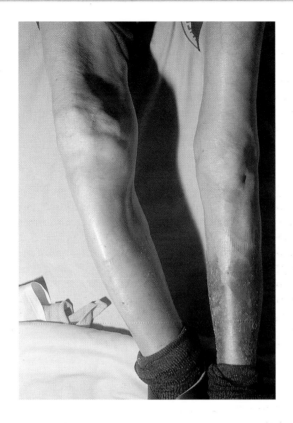

Questions

This patient was deaf.

(a) Name two abnormalities in this photograph.

(b) What is the diagnosis?

(c) Suggest a probable cause of his deafness.

Answers

(a) Bowing of the right tibia and femur, and varicose eczema on the left lower leg.
(b) Paget's disease of bone.
(c) Deafness is due to Paget's disease of the skull – compression of the VIIIth cranial nerve in its cranial canal and pagetic involvement of the ear ossicles.

Short Case (see case 83)

As well as deformity there may be an increased temperature (due to increased blood flow) and tenderness over the area (see case 83). Varicose eczema is due to prolonged venous insufficiency causing haemosiderin staining of the skin.

CASE 93

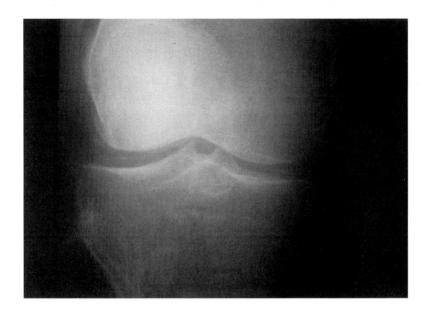

Questions

(a) What is the abnormality in this photograph?

(b) What is the diagnosis?

(c) How is this confirmed?

(d) Name three diseases associated with this condition.

229

Answers

(a) Chondrocalcinosis (obvious in the medial joint compartment).
(b) Pseudogout.
(c) Synovial fluid contains calcium pyrophosphate crystals which are rod or brick shaped and are positively birefringent under polarized light.
(d) Paget's disease, acromegaly, haemochromatosis, hypothyroidism, hyperparathyroidism, diabetes mellitus and Wilson's disease.

Short Case

The knee is the most common joint involved. It results in a swollen knee with an effusion (patella tap). The differential diagnosis is rheumatoid arthritis, osteoarthrosis, gout, septic arthritis, trauma and haemarthrosis secondary to a coagulopathy.

Discussion

Pseudogout is more common in males (2:1) and can be familial. It may occur secondary to other arthropathies such as rheumatoid arthritis, osteoarthrosis and Charcot's joints.

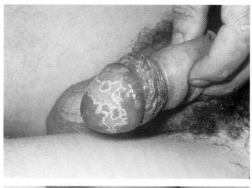

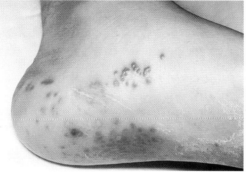

Questions

This 30-year-old man complained of a swollen right ankle.

(a) What two physical signs are shown?

(b) What other symptoms may he have (list two)?

(c) What is the diagnosis?

(d) What is the treatment?

Answers

(a)   Circinate balanitis and keratoderma blenorrhagica.
(b)   Painful/gritty eyes (conjunctivitis and iritis), dysuria and frequency (urethritis), mouth ulcers and backache (sacroiliitis).
(c)   *Reiter's disease.
(d)   Urethritis may respond to tetracycline. Circinate balanitis rarely requires treatment but steroid creams help. Extensive keratoderma responds to systemic steroids. The arthritis responds to non-steroidal anti-inflammatory drugs.

Discussion

Reiter's disease usually affects young men. There is usually a history of sexual intercourse 2 weeks previously. It may also follow bacillary dysentery. It consists of a triad of urethritis, conjunctivitis and arthritis (asymmetrical, usually large joints, lower limbs). Sacroiliitis occurs in 30%. Keratoderma blenhorrhagica occurs in 10% and may be severe, affecting all the body, but occurs most commonly on the soles of the feet followed by the palms of the hands. There may be thickening, ridging and opacity of the nails. Mouth ulceration occurs in 15% of cases. Circinate balanitis occurs in 25% of cases. Subjects with HLA-B27 are more susceptible (present in 70% of cases). The differential diagnosis is: gonoccocal arthritis, ankylosing spondylitis, Behçet's syndrome, psoriatic arthritis and rheumatoid arthritis. Rheumatoid factor is negative. The disease is self limiting but can recur.

***H.C. Reiter** (1881–1969). German professor of hygiene.

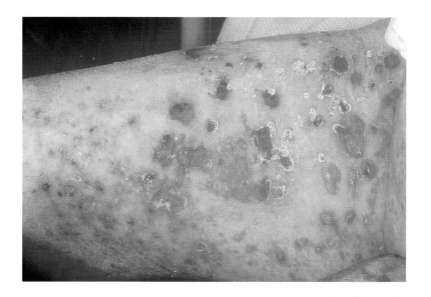

Questions

This 55-year-old woman complained of mouth ulcers. She described 'blisters' on her arms. Her full blood count revealed an eosinophilia and leucocytosis.

(a) What is the diagnosis?

(b) What is the pathology?

(c) What is the treatment?

(d) Name a drug that may cause this condition.

Answers

(a) Pemphigus vulgaris.
(b) The bullae form in the epidermis (in contrast to dermatitis hepatiformis and pemphigoid where bullae are subepidermal). Acantholysis (detachment of epidermal cells from each other) is present (it is absent in the other two bullous disorders). Immunological studies show deposits of IgG in the skin.
(c) Steroids and azathioprine or methotrexate.
(d) Penicillamine, rifampicin and phenylbutazone.

Discussion

Pemphigus occurs in the middle-aged and sexes are equally affected. The blisters occur anywhere on the body and are fragile. Occasionally lesions may occur without initial blister formation. The mucous membranes are commonly affected. It is more common in Jewish people and there is an increased incidence in patients with thymoma and myasthenia gravis.

Acantholysis is the characteristic histological feature and Nikolsky's sign is present (firm pressure exerted on normal skin causes it to slide off).

Treatment requires high-dose prednisolone (100–200 mg daily) initially and azathioprine as a steroid-sparing agent is used. Lesions sometimes become secondarily infected. Without treatment this condition is rapidly fatal.

Pemphigoid is a bullous disorder of the elderly where the bullae are subepidermal and therefore thicker and less likely to rupture than in pemphigus. Mucosal lesions are uncommon and Nikolsky's sign is negative. It may be associated with an underlying malignancy, frusemide, clonididine or PUVA. It is treated with systemic steroids and, unlike pemphigus, does not have a significant mortality.

CASE 96

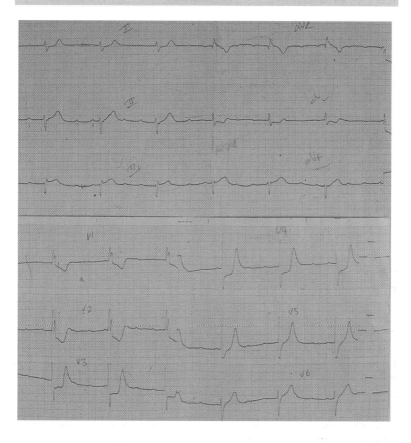

Questions

(a) Name two abnormalities on this ECG.

(b) Name two symptoms the patient may have.

(c) What is the likely cause of the ECG appearance?

Answers

(a) Mobitz type II heart block (2:1 see lead II). It is usually due to impaired conduction in the bundle of His or bundle branches and, therefore, there is usually a broadened QRS complex. There is evidence of right bundle branch block and ST depression in the chest leads. The QRS frontal axis is $-90°$.

(b) Chest pain, dyspnoea (due to heart failure) and dizziness.

(c) Myocardial infarction/ischaemic heart disease.

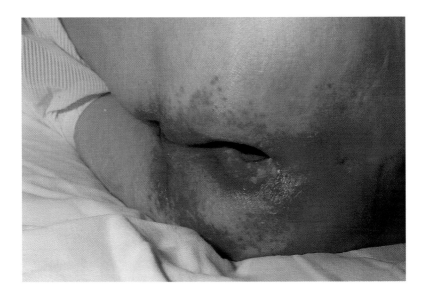

Questions

(a) Name two abnormalities in this photograph.

(b) Name two other areas where it may occur.

Answers

(a) There is a grade IV sacral pressure sore. There is cutaneous candidiasis (note classical satellite lesions).

(b) Areas of bony prominences, e.g. heel, thoracic spine, greater trochanter, ischial tuberosity.

Short Case (see Appendix, Figure 23)

Those at risk include patients with decreased mobility and in the examination situation this may involve a chronic neurological condition, e.g. paraplegia, motor neurone disease, multiple sclerosis or stroke. Be aware of the possibility of pressure sores in these patients.

Discussion

The prevalence of pressure sores is 4–10% of hospitalized patients. Risk factors include old age, immobility (fractures, osteoarthritis, neurological disease), malnutrition, arterial disease and sensory impairment. Many risk factor assessment scales have been developed to determine how 'at risk' some people are, e.g. Waterlow score, Norton. Pressure sores can be classified simply as follows;

- **Grade I** – erythema, skin intact.
- **Grade II** – skin loss, epidermis/dermis (abrasion/blister, shallow crater).
- **Grade III** – full-thickness loss and damage to subcutaneous tissues.
- **Grade IV** – extensive destruction, tissue necrosis or damage to underlying muscle or bone.

Management consists of prevention (awareness of risk factors, special mattresses). In those who have sores; relieve pressure, improve health and nutrition (high calorie intake, more than 2000 kcal per day), clean wound with simple dressings and treat infection with systemic antibiotics.

Pressure sores have a significant morbidity and mortality. They are under reported. They cost the National Health Service approximately £200m annually.

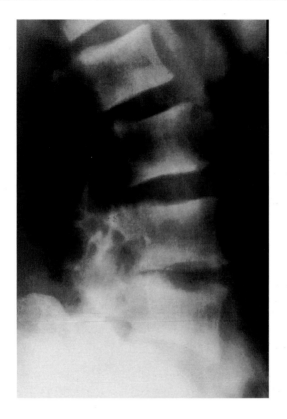

Questions

(a) What is this physical sign?

(b) What is the cause?

Answers

(a) 'Rugger jersey' spine. The end plates are relatively more dense than the rest of the vertebral body giving a 'rugger jersey' appearance.

(b) Renal osteodystrophy. Osteomalacia and secondary hyperparathyroidism (and possibly tertiary hyperparathyroidism) co-exist in chronic renal failure (see case 84). There is a low serum calcium, decreased calcium absorption, hyperphosphataemia, increased alkaline phosphatase and increased plasma parathyroid hormone (calcium may be increased if there is tertiary hyperparathyroidism).

Short Case

Clinical signs of uraemia include: pallor (anaemia is usually normochromic normocytic), skin bruising, brown line near the end of the finger nails, hypertension and its consequences (cardiac failure), hypotension, hyperventilation (Kussmaul's respiration), peripheral neuropathy and palpable kidneys if polycystic disease is present. Pericarditis, muscular twitching, hiccups and uraemic frost (see case 45) are late manifestations in renal failure.

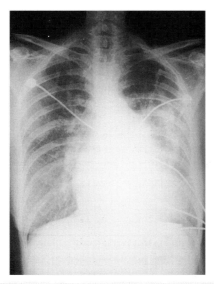

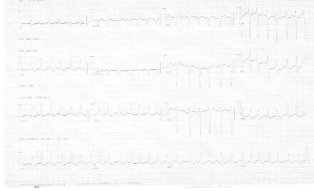

Questions

This patient had splenomegaly and microscopic haematuria.

    (a) Name two abnormalities on the chest X-ray.

    (b) What does the ECG show?

    (c) What is the most likely structural lesion?

    (d) What is the cause of the physical signs?

    (e) What may be seen on fundoscopy in this patient?

Answers

(a) Large left atrium and pulmonary artery (straight left heart border), pulmonary oedema and calcification of the pleura.
(b) Atrial fibrillation. There is ST depression owing to ischaemia resulting from the fast ventricular rate.
(c) Mitral stenosis (see case 62).
(d) Bacterial endocarditis.
(e) A *Roth spot (oval retinal haemorrhage with pale central area). They occur in 5% of cases and may also be seen in systemic lupus erythematosis.

Short Case

There may be finger clubbing, splinter haemorrhages, *Osler's nodes (painful indurated lesions on finger pads), *Janeway's lesions (reddish eruptions on the palms and soles which are nodular and slightly tender, and they fade like a bruise), pallor, fever, splenomegaly and café-au-lait spots (late manifestation). A heart murmur of mitral stenosis will be present (see case 62) and regurgitant murmurs may be heard owing to valve damage. The urine will show microscopic haematuria caused by associated glomerulonephritis.

Discussion

The infecting organisms are *Streptococcus viridans* (45%), *Staphylococcus aureus* and *Staphylococcus albus* (25%), *Streptococcus faecalis* (7%) and others (23%), *Gonococcus, Brucella, Proteus, Coxiella Burneti,* fungi.

There is usually an abnormal valve but healthy valves may be affected (50% of cases) especially in intravenous drug addicts when a normal tricuspid valve may become involved. Ventricular septal defects, patent ductus arteriosus, coarctation of the aorta and biscuspid aortic valves may be affected. Secundum atrial septal defects do not develop endocarditis. Mitral valves are more likely than aortic valves to become involved and regurgitant mitral valves are more susceptible than stenotic ones.

If suspected, at least six blood cultures should be taken. Mortality is about 30%. Death is usually from heart failure, valve destruction or major emboli (cerebral).

Management should include prophylaxis for patients with valve lesions. If the diagnosis is suspected the patient should receive intravenous benzylpenicillin and gentamycin until microbial information is available. If all six blood cultures are negative, consider:
- Unusual organisms – Q fever, Bacteroides, fungi.
- Partly treated cases at presentation.
- *Libman–Sacks endocarditis (non-infective endocarditis of mitral

and/or aortic valves seen in systemic lupus erythematosus but also can occur in polyarteritis nodosa).

- Atrial myxoma.
- Right-sided endocarditis.
- Non-bacterial endocarditis associated with carcinomatosis.

*__M. Roth__ (1839–1914). Swiss pathologist.

*__Sir W. Osler__ (1849–1919). Canadian professor of medicine (see case 74)

*__E.G. Janeway__ (1841–1911). American physician.

*__E. Libman__ (1872–1946). American physician.

*__B. Sacks__ (1873–1939). American physician.

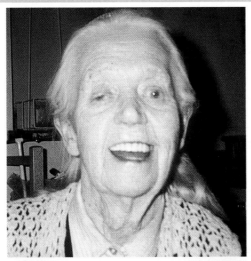

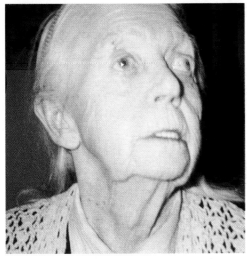

Questions

(a) What is the diagnosis?

(b) List three possible causes.

Answers

(a) Partial right IIIrd cranial nerve palsy.

(b) Aneurysm of the posterior communicating artery (commonest cause), midbrain vascular lesion (if there is contralateral hemiplegia it is due to a lesion at the IIIrd nerve nucleus and cerebral peduncle – *Weber's syndrome), causes of mononeuritis multiplex (see case 6), meningovascular syphilis, carcinomas of the skull base, and encephalitis.

Short Case (see Appendix, Figure 24)

There is ptosis, which may be partial or complete and the nerve palsy is classified by this. The eye is down and out (divergent strabismus). She is unable to look to her left. When the condition is partial (partial ptosis) the patient complains of diplopia (cover test – see case 6).

The pupil is dilated (mydriasis).

*H.D. Weber (1823–1918). German physician.

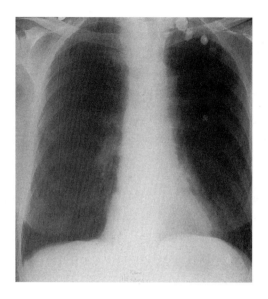

Questions

(a) What abnormality can be seen on this chest X-ray?

(b) What is the cause?

Answers

(a) Calcified foci in the left upper zone.
(b) 'Old' tuberculous infection.

Short Case (see Appendix, Figure 25)

See case 90.

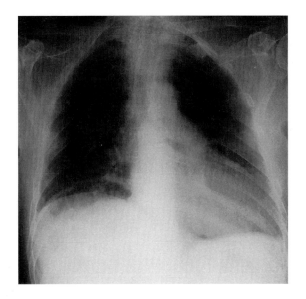

Questions

(a) What abnormality can be seen on this chest X-ray?

(b) What symptoms may the patient have?

(c) What physical sign is significant?

(d) What is the name of this syndrome?

Answers

(a) There is interposition of the colon in front of and above the liver. The haustrations in the colon can be seen below the right hemidiaphragm.

(b) Usually asymptomatic but may have abdominal pain and nocturnal vomiting.

(c) There is loss of liver dullness and bowel sounds in the right upper quadrant.

(d) *Chilaiditi syndrome. The condition was described in 1910 and is more common in children and the elderly.

*D. Chilaiditi. German radiologist.

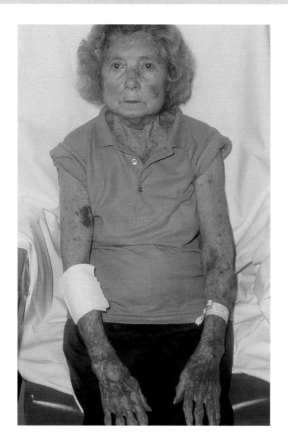

Questions

This woman has asthma.

(a) Name three abnormalities in this photograph.

(b) What is the diagnosis?

(c) What other complications may she have?

Answers

(a) Purpura, thin skin and moon face. Also incidental Bouchard's nodes are seen resulting from osteoarthrosis.

(b) Cushing's syndrome. Due to prolonged use of steroids to control her asthma.

(c) Other complications include osteoporosis, hypertension, diabetes mellitus, poor healing skin, renal stones, depression and mania.

Short Case

See case 76.

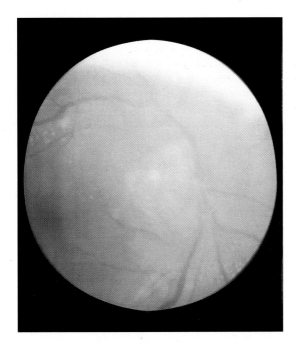

Questions

(a) Name two abnormalities on this fundus.

(b) What is the diagnosis?

(c) List three causes.

Answers

(a)   Soft exudates and papilloedema.

(b)   Malignant ('accelerated') hypertension.

(c)   Causes of her hypertension are:
   (i) **Essential** (idiopathic) – 90% of cases.
   (ii) **Secondary** – 10% of cases:
   – Renal disease (renal artery stenosis, polycystic kidney, pyelonephritis).
   – Endocrine (Cushing's disease, Conn's syndrome, phaeochromocytoma, acromegaly, hyperparathyroidism, hypothyroidism).
   – Others (acute intermittent porphyria, polycythaemia rubra vera, raised intracranial pressure, coactation of the aorta).

Short Case

Hypertensive retinopathy is graded as follows:

- **Grade I** – narrowing of arterioles.
- **Grade II** – copper wiring of arterioles and AV nipping.
- **Grade III** – haemorrhages (usually flame shaped) and exudates (hard or soft; soft implies area of oedema due to rapid increase in blood pressure, hard exudates near the macula can cause a star-like configuration).
- **Grade IV** – Grade III plus papilloedema.

Papilloedema causes enlargement of the blind spot and constriction of the peripheral field but visual acuity is not affected. This must be distinguished from papillitis (optic neuritis) which causes a central scotoma, decreased visual acuity and tenderness and pain on eye movement.

If the hypertension is secondary the patient may have relevant clinical signs, e.g. Cushing's disease, acromegaly or hypothyroidism.

Discussion

The presence of exudates with papilloedema indicates malignant hypertension. The mortality is high if untreated. An underlying cause should be sought. Other causes of papilloedema include:

- Space occupying intracranial lesion – tumour, abscess, haematoma.
- Meningitis/encephalitis.
- Hypercapnoea (cyanosis, flapping tremor).
- Cavernous sinus thrombosis (follows infection of nose, face and orbit, eyeball protrudes and is painful and immobile).
- Hypoparathyroidism (cataracts, tetany).
- Benign intracranial hypertension. Commoner in young women. Associated with the oral contraceptive pill, steroid use, head injury, menarche and pregnancy.

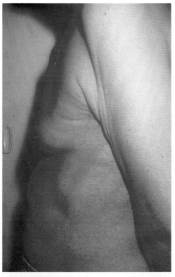

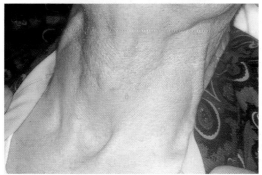

Questions

This 58-year-old man complained of chest tenderness. He had had a myocardial infarction 3 years previously.

(a) What two physical signs are shown?

(b) What is the most likely cause of his chest tenderness?

(c) Name two other causes of this condition.

Answers

(a) Gynaecomastia and a raised jugular venous pressure.

(b) It is most likely that he has developed heart failure due to his previous history of ischaemic heart disease and has been treated with spironolactone and/or digoxin, both of which can cause gynaecomastia.

(c) Causes of gynaecomastia include: senility, liver disease, thyrotoxicosis, hypothyroidism, pituitary disease (hypopituitarism, acromegaly), Addison's disease, a renal carcinoma, testicular carcinoma, carcinoma of the lung, Klinefelter's syndrome (47XXY, small testes, mental deficiency, increased luteinizing hormone (LH) and and follicle-stimulating hormone (FSH)), drugs (oestrogens, digoxin, spironolactone, tricyclic antidepressants, phenothiazines and Cimetidine).

Short Case

Gynaecomastia may be unilateral. Palpate for the presence of breast tissue. Note any other related physical signs such as clubbing (bronchial carcinoma, liver disease), jaundice and spider naevi (chronic liver disease), absence of body hair (hypopituitarism) and increased pigmentation (Addison's disease, liver disease).

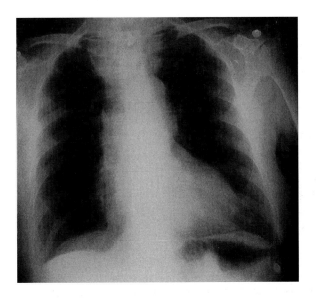

Questions

This female patient complained of dysphagia, constipation and weight gain.

(a) What is the abnormality on this chest X-ray?

(b) What is the most likely diagnosis?

(c) What is the cause of her symptoms?

Answers

(a)   A superior mediastinal mass.

(b)   Retrosternal goitre (dull to percussion).

(c)   Dysphagia is caused by pressure from the goitre. Her symptoms are due to hypothyroidism.

Discussion

Examples of mediastinal masses are as follows:

- **Superior** – goitre, dermoid cyst, thymoma, teratoma.
- **Middle** – hiatus hernia, bronchogenic or pleuropericardial cysts.
- **Posterior** – aortic aneurysm, neurogenic tumours (neurilemmoma, neurofibroma, ganglioneuroma, neuroblastoma).

Causes of mediastinal lymphadenopathy, which is most commonly in the middle and superior mediastinum, include metastatic tumours, lymphomas, sarcoidosis (bilateral and asymptomatic) and primary tuberculosis (local parenchymal lesion).

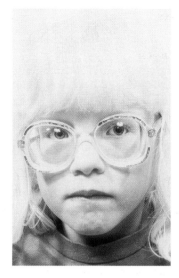
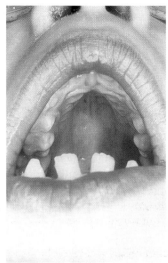

Questions

(a) What two physical signs are apparent?

(b) What is the diagnosis?

(c) Name two other ocular complications.

(d) What is the cause of this condition?

(e) How is the diagnosis confirmed?

(f) What is the inheritance pattern?

Answers

(a) Spectacles because of myopia (uncommon at this age) and a high arched palate is apparent.
(b) Homocystinuria.
(c) Lens dislocation (usually downwards), caused by weakening of the suspensory ligaments, results in iridodonesis (tremor of the iris), glaucoma, myopia and cataracts. Optic atrophy and retinal detachment can occur.
(d) Cystathionine synthase deficiency. This causes an accumulation of homocysteine which is oxidized to homocystine.
(e) Homocystine in urine gives a positive reaction with cyanide nitroprusside reagent and urinary amino acid analysis confirms the diagnosis.
(f) Autosomal recessive.

Short Case

About 50% of patients have mental retardation (15% have fits). Subjects are tall with arachnodactyly, high arched palate, kyphoscoliosis, flat feet, pectus excavatum, hyperextensile joints as a result of lax ligaments (see case 50) and poor muscle development. There is generalized osteoporosis, a malar flush and livedo reticularis.

Discussion

It is treated with dietary restriction of methionine cystine and pyridoxine supplementation. Treatment needs to be started at birth. Women should not take the oral contraceptive pill as there is an increased risk of arterial thromboembolism and there is also a risk during general anaesthetic if the patient has not been treated as stated.

This disease has many features similar to Marfan's syndrome but the two conditions should be distinguished. The features of Marfan's syndrome are: autosomal dominant, tall, high arched palate, arachnodactyly, lens dislocation (and complications), kyphoscoliosis, pectus excavatus, hyperextile joints (see case 50), aortic regurgitation, aortic coarctation, mitral valve prolapse and cystic lung disease (spontaneous pneumothoraces).

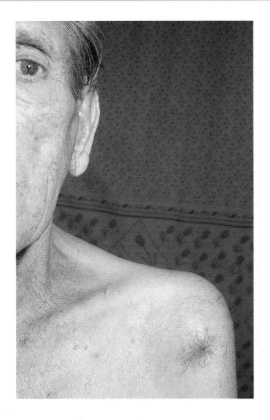

Questions

This 70-year-old man presented with a massive haematemesis.

(a) What physical sign can be seen?

(b) Name two causes of this physical sign.

(c) What is the cause in this case?

(d) What is the most likely cause of his haematemesis?

Answers

(a) Spider naevus (telangiectasia). Central arterial dot from which radiates several dilated vessels which are obliterated by central pressure.
(b) Chronic liver disease, pregnancy and hyperthyroidism. Spider naevi usually occur in the distribution of the superior vena cava (head, neck, chest and upper limbs).
(c) Hepatic cirrhosis.
(d) Oesophageal varices (alcoholics also have a high incidence of peptic ulcers).

Short Case

Look for other signs of chronic liver disease (see cases 37 and 53).

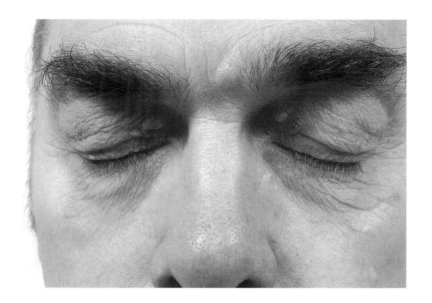

Questions

(a) What is the abnormality?

(b) What is the cause?

(c) What other eye signs may be present?

(d) Name two associated diseases.

(e) What is the treatment?

Answers

(a) Xanthelasma on both upper eye lids.
(b) Hyperlipidaemia (most likely mixed hyperlipidaemia, type IIb; cholesterol and triglycerides are both elevated).
(c) Corneal arcus.
(d) Hypertension, diabetes mellitus and ischaemic heart disease.
(e) Low fat diet (polyunsaturated fats are substituted), low sugar and alcohol, stop smoking and control hypertension. If there is no reduction in the lipids, oral agents may be needed, e.g. Bezafibrate.

Discussion

Frederickson's classification of hyperlipoproteinaemia is as follows.

Types IIa, IIb and IV are the most common.
- **Type IIa** – familial hypercholesterolaemia (high cholesterol, normal triglyceride level).
  Commoner in females.
  Primary or secondary to hypothyroidism, cholestatic jaundice and nephrotic syndrome.
  Corneal arcus, tendens xanthomata (Achilles) and tuberous xanthomata (extensor surfaces). Associated with early ischaemic heart disease.
- **Type IIb** – mixed hyperlipidaemia (increased cholesterol and increased triglyceride). Associated with ischaemic heart disease, hypothyroidism and diabetes mellitus. Xanthelasma, corneal arcus.
- **Type IV** – hypertriglyceridaemia (cholesterol level normal or high).
  Commoner in females.
  Primary or secondary to diabetes mellitus and obesity.
  Associated with gout, alcoholism and pancreatitis.
  Causes early ischaemic heart disease and hypertension.
  Eruptive cutaneous xanthomata.

The following are rare:
- **Type I** – hyperchylomicronaemia – xanthomata and pancreatitis.
- **Type II** – increased cholesterol, increased triglycerides. Fat deposition in palm creases.
- **Type V** – combined I and IV.

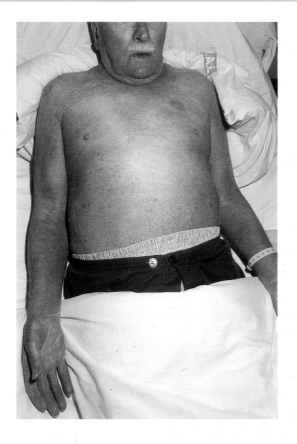

Questions

This 76-year-old man complained of thirst and pruritus for 2 days. He had been commenced on an antidepressant 3 days previously.

(a) What is the diagnosis?

(b) What is the cause?

(c) Name two other causes of this condition.

(d) What is the cause of his thirst?

Answers

(a) Erythroderma ('exfoliative dermatitis').
(b) Drug allergy.
(c) Eczema, psoriasis, lymphoma and leukaemia.
(d) Dehydration resulting from increased insensible loss through dilated skin vessels.

Discussion

Erythroderma is the term applied to inflammatory skin disease that affects more than 90% of the body surface. There is often a widespread oedema and facial oedema which may result in conjunctivitis. The condition has a mortality owing to its systemic effect and pneumonia and heart failure are the most common causes of death. Other systems affected include:

- **Haemodynamic effects** – increased cardiac output, increased plasma volume, oedema, collapsing pulse, increased blood flow to the skin and decreased flow to other organs.
- **Thermoregulation** – fluctuation in body temperature. Hypothermia in cold rooms because of inability to vasoconstrict skin vessels. Hyperpyrexia in hot rooms due to increased metabolic rate. Inappropriate shivering occurs.
- **Haematological effects** – anaemia (due to malabsorption), folate deficiency, leucocytosis, increased ESR, hypoalbuminaemia, increased plasma globulins.
- **Malabsorption** – reversible by treating erythroderma and also there may be a protein-losing enteropathy ('dermatogenic enteropathy').
- **Lymphadenopathy**
- **Hypocalcaemia** – secondary to hypoalbuminaemia or malabsorption.
- **Others** – gynaecomastia and hyperuricaemia in erythrodermic psoriasis owing to increased cell turnover.

Treatment consists of topical steroids but systemic steroids may be necessary. Other treatments are supportive, e.g. intravenous fluids if dehydrated, and treatment of heart failure.

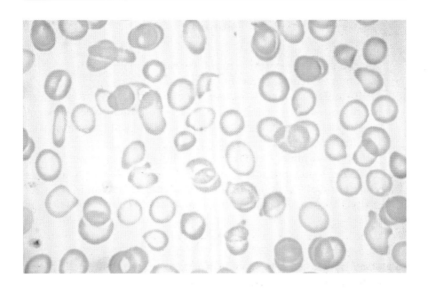

Questions

(a) What are the abnormalities on this peripheral blood film?

(b) What is the diagnosis?

(c) Name three possible causes.

(d) Name three physical signs the patient may have.

CASE 111

Answers

(a)   Red cells are microcytic and hypochromic and there are pencil-shaped poikilocytes (there may be occasional target cells).

(b)   Severe iron deficiency anaemia.

(c)   This can be classified as follows:

    (i) **Blood loss** – menorrhagia, gastrointestinal bleed (ulcers, varices, carcinoma), haematuria (renal/bladder carcinomas).

    (ii) **Increased demand** – pregnancy.

    (ii) **Malabsorption** – coeliac disease, inflammatory bowel disease, blind loop syndrome.

    (iv) **Poor diet** – common in the elderly and vegetarians.

(d)   Pallor, brittle nails, koilonychia, glossitis and angular stomatitis.

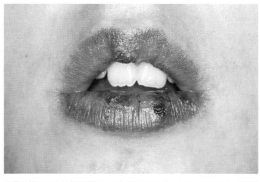

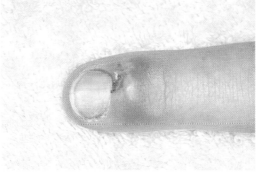

Questions

This 16-year-old girl had a temperature of 38°C.

(a) What are the lesions shown?

(b) What is the cause?

(c) How is the diagnosis made?

(d) What is the treatment?

CASE 112

Answers

(a) Herpetic stomatitis and herpetic whitlow.
(b) Herpes Simplex type I virus (type II causes genital herpes).
(c) Isolation of the virus from lesions and a rising antibody level.
(d) Symptomatic: analgesics, antipyretics and mouth washes. Acyclovir in the early stages is effective. Local application of 40% idoxuridine is helpful for the whitlow.

Discussion

Herpetic stomatitis is the most common manifestation of herpes simplex particularly in young children. The onset is with fever and malaise. Vesicles appear around the mouth and the mouth is sore. There may also be discrete lesions on the face, trunk and limbs. The mouth lesions are ulcers with a white exudate which bleed when touched. There is an associated lymphadenopathy. After the initial infection the viruses lie dormant in the dorsal root ganglia. From time to time a stimulus (pneumonia, cold, trauma, fatigue, strong sunlight, pre-menstrual) causes reactivation of the virus with the formation of new lesions ('cold sores'). The primary infection is sometimes subclinical and the first apparent infection is a cold sore. This lesion is highly infectious and is spread by kissing. The differential diagnosis of stomatitis includes: aphthous stomatitis, herpangina, hand-foot and mouth disease, Stevens–Johnson syndrome, a granulocytosis, SLE, pemphigus and Vincent's stomatitis.

A herpetic whitlow is a true viral wound infection. Surgical incision should be avoided as the condition is self-limiting.

Other clinical manifestations of herpes infection include:

- Generalized infection of the newborn. Type II virus, which is rare and usually acquired from the mother who is suffering from genital herpes. It is frequently fatal.
- Keratoconjunctivitis. This presents with conjunctivitis and is usually unilateral. It may lead to dendritic ulcers and damage the vision.
- Genital herpes. Type II virus. Sexually transmitted disease. This may play a role in cervical cancer.
- Eczema herpeticum (Kaposi's varicelliform eruption). In patients with eczema, primary infection of the skin can cause serious illness with widespread vesicles. The illness may be fatal.
- Herpes encephalitis. Rare. This presents with cerebral irritation, convulsions and impaired consciousness. Oedema may cause localized signs. Mortality is high (60%).

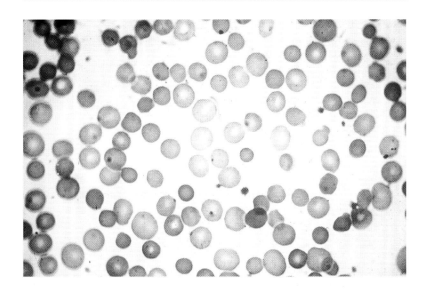

Questions

This patient complained of right upper quadrant pain.

(a) Describe the abnormalities on this blood film.

(b) What is the diagnosis?

(c) What is the inheritance pattern?

(d) Name three possible physical signs.

(e) What is the probable cause of the patient's right upper quadrant pain?

Answers

(a) Microspherocytes can be seen that are densely staining and have smaller diameters than normal red cells.
(b) Hereditary spherocytosis
(c) Autosomal dominant (variable expression).
(d) Pallor (anaemia), jaundice (secondary to haemolysis) and splenomegaly.
(e) Gallstones (pigment stones are common).

Discussion

Hereditary spherocytosis is the most common haemolytic anaemia in Northern Europeans. Haemolytic anaemia may be classified as:

- **Hereditary** – Red cell membrane disorder, e.g. hereditary spherocytosis, hereditary elliptocytosis.
  - Red cell metabolism defect, e.g. G6PD deficiency, pyruvate kinase deficiency.
  - Red cell haemoglobin defect, e.g. abnormal haemoglobin (HbS, HbC), defective synthesis, e.g. thalassaemia.
- **Acquired**
  - Immune.
  - Hypersplenism.
  - Secondary to renal/liver failure.
  - Paroxysmal nocturnal haemoglobinuria.
  - Others: infections, toxins, chemicals, drugs.

Clinical features of haemolysis are anaemia, jaundice and splenomegaly. There is excess urobilinogen in the urine which turns dark on standing. Pigment gallstones occur. Aplastic crises are usually precipitated by infection. Folate deficiency is common because of the increased cell turnover. Laboratory findings are as follows:

- Increased red cell breakdown (increased bilirubin, increased urinary urobilinogen, increased faecal stercobilinogen, decreased serum haptoglobulins).
- Increased red cell production (reticulocytosis, erythroid hyperplasia of bone marrow).
- Damaged red cells (fragments, osmotic fragility, decreased red cell survival as shown by the ^{51}Cr labelling test).

In hereditary spherocytosis the marrow produces red cells of the normal biconcave shape but these lose membrane as they circulate through the spleen and reticuloendothelial system. The spherocytes produced are unable to pass through the splenic circulation and die early.

The treatment is splenectomy. It should be avoided in young children because of the increased risk of pneumococcal infection. Folic acid supplements must be given. Pneumococcal vaccination must be given before splenectomy.

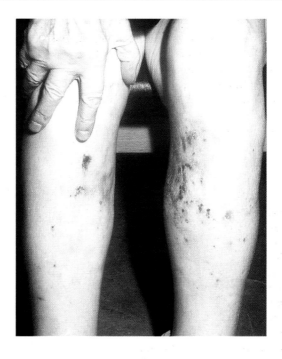

Questions

This 80-year-old woman is housebound and lives alone. She has difficulty getting out of a chair and perioral paraesthesiae.

(a) What can be seen in the photograph?

(b) What is the probable cause?

(c) What other signs may she have?

(d) What is the cause of her symptoms?

Answers

(a) Petechial haemorrhages on the shins.
(b) Scurvy.
(c) Results in perifollicular haemorrhages, bruises, mucosal haemorrhages (bleeding gums), gum hypertrophy (see case 52) and haemarthroses.
(d) These are due to proximal myopathy and hypocalcaemia caused by associated osteomalacia (see case 75).

Short Case

The patient is undernourished owing to a poor diet. Look for cachexia, anaemia (pallor, glossitis) and bruising, which is due to vitamin C and vitamin K deficiency. There may be oedema resulting from hypoproteinaemia. Bone tenderness, proximal myopathy and tetany (Trousseau's and Chvostek's signs) may be present as a result of osteomalacia (see case 75). Signs of subacute combined degeneration of the spinal cord (weakness, hypertonia, hyperreflexia, extensor plantar responses, loss of vibration and position sensation) and peripheral neuropathy caused by B12 deficiency is very rare in association with a poor diet.

Discussion

Dietary deficiencies may be severe in the elderly especially those who live alone. The treatment is to improve the diet with the addition of necessary supplements initially. A similar picture of malnutrition may of course be due to a malabsorption syndrome (coeliac disease is not uncommon in the elderly) but the patient may have other symptoms prompting this diagnosis, which will require further investigation (diarrhoea, nausea, steatorrhoea, abdominal pain, abdominal distension).

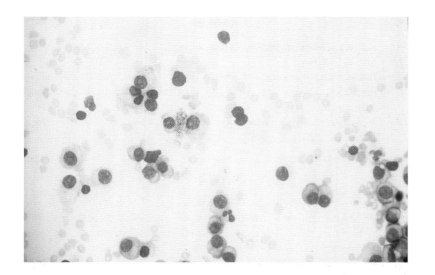

Questions

(a) What does this bone aspirate show?

(b) What is the diagnosis?

(c) List three complications.

(d) Name two drugs used in the treatment.

Answers

(a) A proliferation of plasma cells.

(b) Multiple myeloma.

(c) Bone pain, anaemia, repeated infections, renal failure, bleeding tendency (thrombocytopenia), carpal tunnel syndrome, amyloidosis and hyperviscosity syndrome.

(d) Melphalan, cylophosphamide.
   (See case 25).

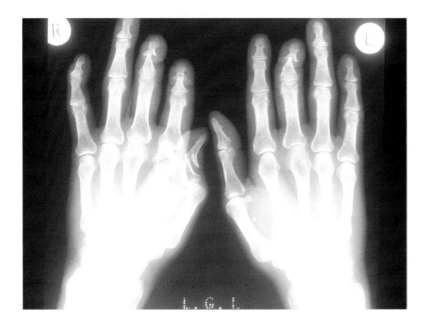

Questions

(a) List three abnormalities on this X-ray.

(b) What is the diagnosis?

(c) List two other physical signs the patient may have.

Answers

(a) Destruction of the DIP joint and distal phalanx of the right index finger. Destruction of the terminal and middle phalanges of the left index and middle fingers. Z-shaped deformity of the left thumb.
(b) Psoriatic arthropathy (arthritis mutilans).
(c) Psoriasis (see case 57), pitting of the nails and onycholysis (see case 71).

Discussion

Psoriatic arthritis may resemble rheumatoid arthritis in 30% of cases. It is seronegative and 30% of patients also have sacroiliitis. The arthritis may be severe and destructive (arthritis mutilans) or it may be an asymmetrical oligo- or monoarthropathy. Non-steroidal anti-inflammatory drugs are the mainstay of treatment. Chloroquine is contra-indicated as it may exacerbate the skin lesions (exfoliative dermatitis). Intra-articular steroids are useful for single inflamed joints. See cases 57 and 71.

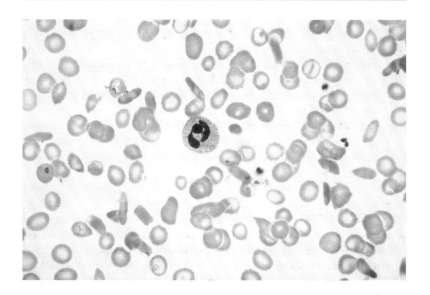

Questions

(a) What can be seen on this blood film and what is the diagnosis?

(b) What is the cause of this disease?

(c) What is the treatment?

CASE 117

Answers

(a) Sickle cells and target cells. Sickle cell anaemia.
(b) Substitution of valine for glutamic acid in position 6 in the beta chain (HbS). HbS is insoluble and forms crystals when exposed to low oxygen tension. Red cells sickle and block different areas of the circulation with resultant infarction.
(c) Avoid the factors that precipitate a crisis, e.g. infection, maintain good nutrition and hygiene. In a crisis: rest, rehydrate, antibiotics, analgesics and correct acidosis. Care is needed in pregnancy and during anaesthesia.

Discussion

Sickle cell anaemia is most prevalent in Central Africa, India and Mediterranean areas. Crises in sickle cell anaemia (homozygous disease, 80–90% of the haemoglobin is abnormal) may be painful, aplastic, haemolytic or infectious. Painful areas are precipitated by infection, hypoxia, dehydration, exercise, cold or childbirth. Infarcts may occur in different organs, e.g. bones, lungs and spleen. Splenic infarcts result in hyposplenism. In children painful dactylitis occurs with resultant deformity of the fingers. Osteomyelitis caused by *Salmonella* may develop in infarcted bones. Renal infarcts cause renal failure. Aplastic crises are caused by infection (especially parvovirus) and there is a sudden drop in the haemoglobin. Ulcers of the legs caused by vascular stasis and ischaemia are common.

Heterozygotes (30% of the haemoglobin is abnormal) have the sickle cell trait in which there is no anaemia but crises occur with severe anoxia or infection.

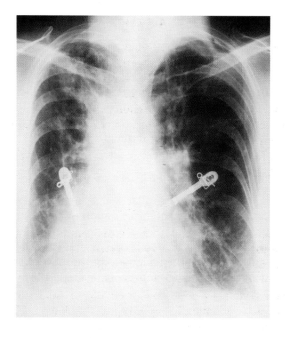

Questions

This 35-year-old man is infertile.

(a) What two abnormalities can be seen on his chest X-ray?

(b) What is the diagnosis?

(c) Name two other associations.

(d) What is the cause of his infertility?

CASE 118

Answers

(a) Chronic bilateral basal lung shadows (due to bronchiectasis) and dextrocardia.
(b) Kartagener's syndrome.
(c) Sinusitis, dysplasia of frontal sinuses, situs inversus and otitis media. There is ciliary immotility resulting in recurrent infection and bronchiectasis.
(d) Immotile sperm (females are fertile).

Short Case

If asked to examine the cardiovascular system the apex beat will not be palpated in the usual position and heart sounds will not be heard on the left. If so, listen to the right thorax for heart sounds. Examine for bronchiectasis (clubbing, bilateral coarse crackles, areas of lung collapse/fibrosis). Examine the abdomen for situs inversus (liver in the left upper quadrant, appendicectomy scar in the left iliac fossa). (See case 20).

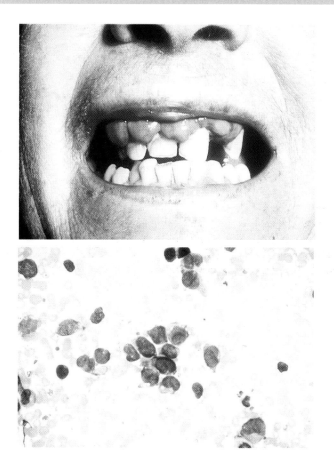

Questions

This bone marrow aspirate belongs to a 28-year-old man.

    (a) What can be seen in the aspirate?

    (b) What is the physical sign shown?

    (c) What is the diagnosis?

Answers

(a)   Proliferation of myeloblasts.
(b)   Gum hypertrophy.
(c)   Acute myelomonocytic leukaemia.

Short Case

Acute leukaemia results in anaemia (pallor), bleeding (petechial haemorrhages and bruises) and infections. There is usually no hepatosplenomegaly in acute myeloid leukaemia.

Discussion

Acute myeloid leukaemia is more common in adults but can occur in children. It can be divided into six variants. Acute myelomonocytic leukaemia (M4 variant) tends to cause tissue deposits (gum hypertrophy, rectal ulceration and skin involvement) and meningeal leukaemia more frequently than the other variants.

The clinical presentation and mortality is due to neutropenia, thrombocytopenia and anaemia caused by bone marrow failure. Clinical features include pallor, anaemia, dyspnoea, fever, mouth, throat and skin infections, bleeding and bruising.

Treatment is supportive and with cytotoxic therapy. The remission rate is 60–80%. The prognosis is poor, the median survival being 12–18 months. Bone marrow transplantation offers the only 'cure'.

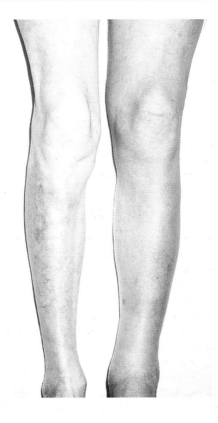

Questions

(a) What is the abnormality shown?

(b) What is the diagnosis?

(c) Name three possible causes.

(d) What abnormalities may be on the ECG?

CASE 120

Answers

(a) Swollen plethoric left leg and thigh.
(b) Iliofemoral deep vein thrombosis (above knee).
(c) Carcinomatosis, post-surgery and oral contraceptives (see case 13).
(d) S1 Q3 T3 pattern, right bundle branch block and atrial fibrillation.

Short Case

The left leg will be swollen and warm to the touch compared with the right. There may be tenderness in the calf and thigh. *Homans' sign may be positive (passive dorsiflexion of the foot causes pain in the calf). This may dislodge clots and is therefore not without danger and should perhaps be discussed but omitted if the diagnosis is obvious.

Discussion

An underlying cause should be sought. A pelvic ultrasound scan is advisable because of possible compression of the pelvic vein in this case.

*J. Homans (1877–1954). American surgeon.

286

Appendix

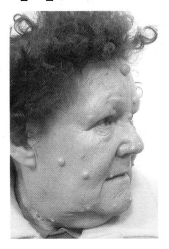

Figure 1 (see case 1). Neurofibromatosis (several neurofibromas can be seen on the face).

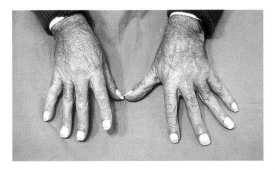

Figure 2 (see case 3). Finger clubbing and leuconychia (due to hypoalbuminaemia) associated with chronic liver disease.

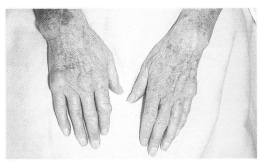

Figure 3 (see case 7). Chronic tophaceous gout.

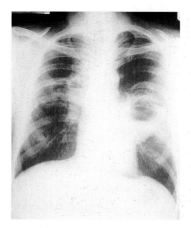

Figure 4 (see case 10).
Lung abscess.

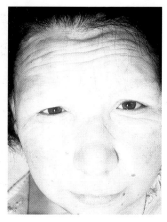

Figure 5 (see case 12).
Hypothyroidism.

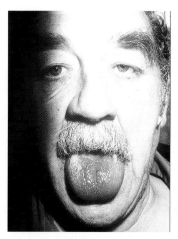

Figure 6 (see case 16). Acromegaly (macroglossia, large nose and jaw).

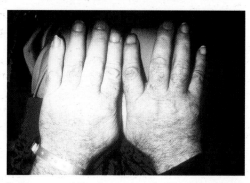

Figure 7 (see case 16). Acromegaly ("spade-like' hands).

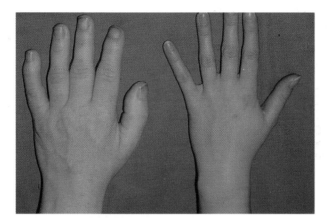

Figure 8 (see case 16). Acromegaly (female patient's hand on the left and the hand of a normal female of similar age on the right).

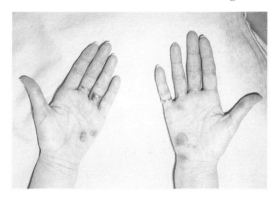

Figure 9 (see case 19). Erythema nodosum on the hands in a patient with Crohn's disease.

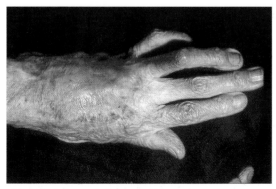

Figure 10 (see case 42). Chronic fibrosis and scarring due to dermatitis artifacta.

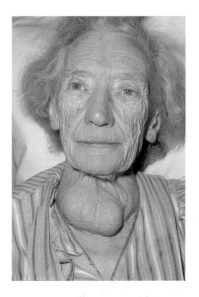

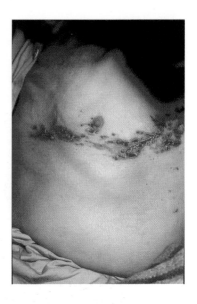

Figure 11 (see case 44).
Multinodular goitre.

Figure 12 (see case 47).
Herpes zoster (shingles)
affecting the left T5
dermatome.

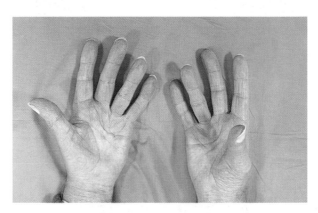

Figure 13 (see case 53). Bilateral Dupuytren's contractures.

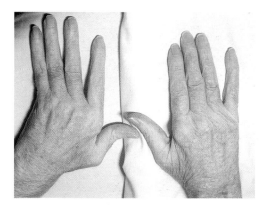

Figure 14 (see case 56). Rheumatoid arthritis showing swollen MCP joints, ulnar deviation in the left hand and Z-shaped deformity of the left thumb.

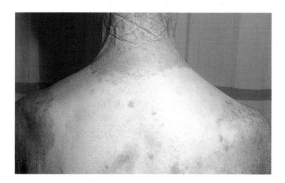

Figure 15 (see case 61). Vitiligo.

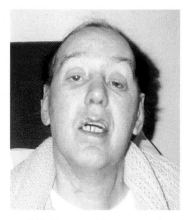

Figure 16 (see case 66). Dystrophia myotonica (frontal balding, bilateral ptosis, transverse smile).

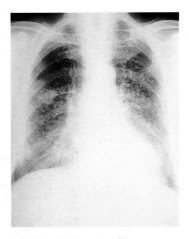

Figure 17 (see case 73). Miliary shadowing.

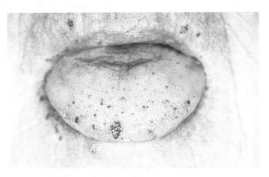

Figure 18 (see case 74). Hereditary haemorrhagic telangiectasia.

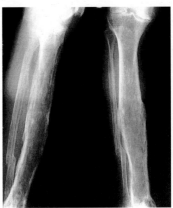

Figure 19 (see case 83). Paget's disease of bone (thickened, disorganized bone, note pathological fracture of fibula).

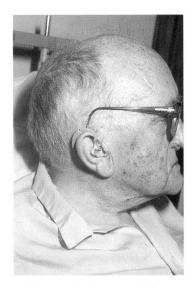

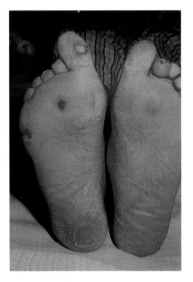

Figure 20 (see case 83).
Paget's disease of skull
(note hearing aid).

Figure 21 (see case 85).
Neuropathic ulcer.

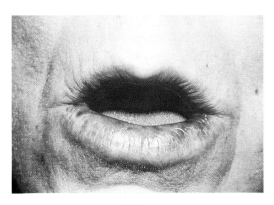

Figure 22 (see case 91). Addison's disease (lip pigmentation).

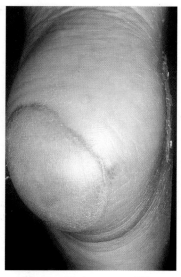

Figure 23 (see case 97).
Bullous lesion on heel due to prolonged pressure.

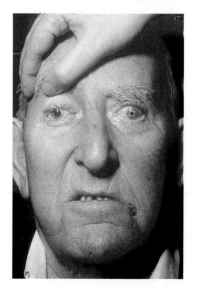

Figure 24 (see case 100).
Left complete IIIrd
cranial nerve palsy.

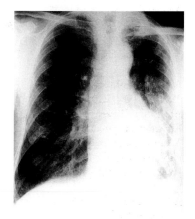

Figure 25 (see case 101).
Left pleural calcification.
Collapse (and chronic
shadowing at the left base
caused by old tuberculous
infection).

INDEX

Numbers in *italics* refer to illustrations

Regurgitation *(continued)*
 tricuspid 7, 64, 72, 108, 136
Reiter's disease *231*, 232
Renal
 adenocarcinoma 76
 artery stenosis 14, *165*, 166
 carcinoma 156
 colic 212
 failure 26, 120, 204, 240, 276
 infarcts 280
 mass, CT scan *19*
 osteodystrophy *239*, 240
 stones 192
Respiratory
 failure, type I 42
 system, examination 8-9
Retinoids 150
Retinopathy
 diabetic *15*, 16, *49*, 50, 170
 hypertensive 166, *253*, 254
Rheumatic fever 54, 160
Rheumatoid arthritis 114, *145*-147,
  184, *291*
Rib notching 14
Rifampicin 224, 234
Rigors 33, 182
Role play in examinations 2, 3
Roth spot 242
Rubeosis iridis 16

Sacroiliitis 150, 232, 278
Sarcoidosis 54, 98, 184, 218
Scalene lymph node 34, 122
Schistosomiasis 218
Scleritis *113*, 114
Sclerodactyly 204
Scleromalacia *113*, 114, 146
Sclerosis, systemic 158, 184, *203*-205
Scurvy 138, *273*, 274
Selegiline 86
Sensation, testing for 12
Serotonin 64-65
Shingles *123*-125
Short case, clinical and oral 2
Shy–Drager syndrome 87
Sickle cell anaemia *279*, 280
Sinemet 86

Sinusitis 142, 282
Sipple's syndrome 20, 94
Sister Mary Joseph nodule *167*, 168
Situs inversus *55*, 56, *281*, 282
Sjögren's syndrome 146, 147
Skin
 appearance, radiotherapy
  treatment *43*
 depigmentation *157*, 158
 flushing *63*, 64
 malar 30, 72
Small cell carcinomas, bronchus
  105, 106
Smell and taste 11
Snoring 67, 68
Soft exudates
 diabetic retinopathy *15*, 16, *49*, 50
 malignant hypertension *253*, 254
Sore throat, streptococcal 54
Spherocytosis, hereditary *271*, 272
Spider naevi 102, *261*, 262
Spinal cord, degeneration 274
Spironolactone 256
Splenomegaly 272
Splinter haemorrhages 242
Steatorrhoea 203
Steele–Richardson syndrome 87
Stokes–Adams attacks 172
Stomach carcinoma *see* Gastric:
  carcinoma
Strabismus *97*, 98, *245*, 246
Streptococcal infection 54, 77, 78
Striae, abdominal *167*, 168, *191*, 192
Stridor 44, 196
Subconjunctival haemorrhages *43*, 44
Subcutaneous
 calcinosis 203, 204
 emphysema 201, 202
Sulphinpyrazone 27
Summarizing findings 6
Superior vena cava obstruction 43,
  44, 106
Supraclavicular lymph nodes 34, 44,
  46, 58, 122
Surgical emphysema *201*, 202
'Swan neck' deformity 146, *179*, 180
Sweating, excessive 48, 116
Syncope 172